The

Gyne's Guide

for

College
Women

The

Gyne's Guide

for

College
Women

How to Have a Healthy,
Safe, and Happy Four Years

A Gynecologist's Perspective

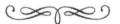

M. SUSAN SCANLON, MD

ScanlonWorks, LLC

The Library of Congress Cataloging-in-Publication Data is available upon request.

ISBN-10: 0996333703
ISBN-13: 978-0-9963337-0-2

Printed in the United States of America
Cover design by Bespoke Book Covers
Author photograph by Papadakis Photography

Although the case studies in this book are real, all names and identifying characteristics have been changed to protect the privacy of the patients.

At the time of this publication, all the facts and statistics cited are the most current available. All website URLs, apps, and phone numbers were active and accurate as of publication. All publications, organizations, websites and other resources existed as described in the guidebook and were verified as of publication. The author and ScanlonWorks, LLC do not warrantee or guarantee the information given out by organizations or content found at websites, and we are not responsible for any changes that occurred after this guidebooks publication.
If you find any error, please contact ScanlonWorks, LLC

This book is written to provide up-to-date information, with accurate and authoritative information about the subject matter covered. It is not intended to substitute for the medical advice from the reader's personal physician, health advisor, or other professional before adopting any of the suggestions in this guidebook or drawing inferences from them. The author and publisher specifically disclaim all responsibility for any liability, loss or risk, personal or otherwise, that is incurred as a consequence, directly or indirectly, of the use or application of any of the contents of this book. The author and ScanlonWorks, LLC disclaim any liability for the decisions you make based on this information.

Author's Note: The Dietary Guidelines for Americans were updated in December 2015 after this book was originally published. To ensure the reader has current nutrition information, this book was updated in April 2016.

10 9 8 7 6 5 4 3 2

First Edition May 2015
Updated April 2016

To my daughters,
≈ Katy & Meghan ≈

You are fabulous young women who
make me so proud!
May you always be healthy and safe
and find happiness in all you do.
Believe in yourselves &
Step confidently forward to tell the
world your message!
xoxo

~ *Contents* ~

Be Happy

Introduction

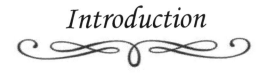

When I set out on my own to go to college, I was on top of the world! Yes, I was a little nervous, but I couldn't wait to forge ahead, move to a new city, and participate in all the freedom and excitement of college life. Soon after starting my freshman year, I realized that although I was confident and academically prepared to take on the schoolwork, I really didn't have a clue about how to take care of myself. Years later, as a doctor to thousands of college girls, I realize that young women, like myself at their age, need more information about the health and social issues they will face in college...and they need it before they leave home.

I grew up in a supportive family and went to a challenging high school. I was not in "the popular group" but had many kind and happy friends. I knew most of the kids in my high school, and although I didn't know all the students personally, I at least knew about them, the values they held, and who their friends were. I felt a sense of comfort and control in knowing everyone.

Most things were scheduled and planned for me during high school. I had a few choices for electives, but generally, the school organized my day. I didn't have to think too much about how to eat healthy because I ate the dinner my mom made and snacked on whatever was in the cabinet. I took dance classes and participated in team sports to stay fit, and the coaches told me what to do.

I did what most other kids were doing—classes, homework, a few after-school activities, and out with friends on the weekends. I followed the schedule and did well. Everything was very predictable. They were all good things, but none of which adequately prepared me for moving out on my own after high school.

When I got to college, nothing was predictable or planned for me. I had to figure it out on my own, and initially I was not very successful. I went to the cafeteria and ate whatever was there without any thought, and I gained weight. I didn't have a coach giving me directions about how far to run or what stretches to do, and so I stopped exercising. I made assumptions that everyone had the same values as the people I knew from home, and I put myself in certain social situations that I was not prepared for and which were really not safe for me. I had more time on my hands in college than in high school, and I found myself out socializing a lot my freshman year, which made it difficult and stressful for me to keep up with my schoolwork, and made me feel "run down." I didn't feel the same sense of control that I had in high school. Wow, I was in for a big surprise when I left home for college, and I really didn't know how to stay on top of it all.

As a gynecologist, I listen to my patients and realize they are experiencing many of the same challenges navigating college as I did. Although they were taught in their high school health classes about a balanced diet, daily exercise, safe sex, avoiding STDs, and risk of alcohol poisoning, many of my patients say they just "tuned out" the information at the time. When faced with the numerous health and social situations in college, many young women are not prepared and end up making unhealthy and unsafe choices.

In addition, I have observed that most of my patients feel uncertain about how to adjust to college and regain a sense of control in their lives away from home. Many make choices that are not consistent with their personal values, just to fit in, and are not as happy as they could be with the outcomes of their decisions.

Learning to handle stress, eat healthy, stay fit, protect yourself, and make choices consistent with the woman you want to be are all important parts of success and happiness in college. I have written this guidebook to help you understand what you will face in college so you can take care of yourself and stay on track to reaching your college goals. The information is very detailed and tells you what to do and the exact steps to take. It can be read all at once, or used as a reference during your college years and beyond.

College can be some of the best years of your life. You will meet many new people and learn an abundance of interesting things. Infinite opportunities are ahead for you! So let's get YOU prepared to move out on your own, be the best you can be, and have the healthiest, safest, and happiest experience in college!

Chapter 1
Getting Prepared:
Four Steps Before College

Congratulations, you're among the thousands of women headed to college this year! All your studying and hard work has paid off... You've taken your opportunity and are making it a reality! This is an exciting time in your life, and you'll want to get a great start to make the next four years the best they can be. Now let's get you prepared!

Here's why...

Guess when the busiest time in my office for college women is? Maybe you've guessed the few weeks before everyone heads out in the fall? No. It's actually two days during Thanksgiving break.

As a gynecologist, I add extra office hours on the Friday and Saturday after Thanksgiving to take care of the women coming home from college with problems. They're usually freshmen. Some office visits are scheduled to treat abnormal periods, weight gain, or yeast infections, while other appointments are to address sexually transmitted diseases, contraception, or sexual assault. I have taken care of thousands of college women during the last 19 years and realize that women need more information before they leave home.

Several books are available to help you organize your dorm room, decide what clothes and supplies to bring, and learn how to tackle some social issues from the perspective of a recent college grad. This book is different in that it's from the perspective of a gynecologist, and it tells you how to prepare YOU! Being prepared will give you the healthiest, safest, and happiest experience in college.

As a doctor, I have seen that the young women who have a solid sense of self, including their personal values, often make the healthiest lifestyle choices in college. They also seem happiest with the outcomes of their decisions.

The most important thing to do in getting ready for college is to think things through BEFORE you go. Give thought to who YOU really are and how to make choices that are in keeping with the best vision of yourself. Advanced planning will help you feel good about the decisions you make and be your healthiest.

Maybe this sounds difficult or confusing, but it doesn't have to be. In the following pages, I have outlined the detailed steps you need to take BEFORE you leave home. Later chapters give you in-depth information about each situation you will face during college and the things you can do to best take care of yourself.

The details in this guidebook will not be sugarcoated, and much of what I talk about can make you feel embarrassed. You're not alone. Who doesn't feel embarrassed about what gynecologists talk about? But, it's what you need to know as a college woman, so I encourage you to read through the chapters in privacy, or talk them over with a trusted friend or family member. Then use this guidebook as a reference during the next four years.

You've worked very hard to get to college. Now, take the time you deserve to understand what's ahead for you and decide how you want to stay on top of it all. Being prepared will help you be your best and tackle problems with confidence. Maybe you're tired of reading books, and just want to get to college? I promise you, reading this guidebook may be the most important homework you've ever done. Now let's get started!

> ## Pre-College Homework Part One:
> ### *Four Steps to Getting Prepared Before Leaving Home*

Step 1. Start by Asking Yourself these Important Questions
- "What kind of woman do I want to be?"
- "What are my boundaries?"

No matter who you are, where you come from, what your family background is, or the hardships you may have faced, you have the ability to choose who you want to be. You get to decide what's important to you and where you want to go in life. You get to choose the woman that you want to be.

Think about who you are now compared to the vision of the woman you want to be...do you need to make any changes? Are your personal values consistent with your vision?

Defining your boundaries and personal values before you move away from home will help you make decisions in college that are consistent with the woman you want to be. Having a solid sense of self will give you the strength and confidence you need to be your best and to take on any challenge that college presents.

Step 2. Set Your Standards High & Choose to Live Up to Them

You have the opportunity to expand on the great qualities you've developed over the last four years as you gain your independence in college. On the other hand, if you've made some choices that weren't the best and you're ready for a change, now is the time!

There will be many distractions in college that can derail you from your path. No one is perfect and everyone makes mistakes, but the goal is to think carefully about your lifestyle choices and to keep trying to be your best. Living up to the standards you've set for yourself may be difficult sometimes, but this approach to college is completely worth the effort and will help you stay on track to reaching your goals.

Step 3. Have a Plan in Advance of Going to College

To get YOU prepared for college, you need to understand the health and social situations that you will face in college, and then plan ahead for how you want to handle them. Understanding your personal values will help you make decisions that you can feel good about. Having a clear plan in mind will help you avoid doing things "just to fit in."

My patients who have had something "go wrong" on their path often feel less upset with the outcome if they made the decision based on their values in the first place. On the other hand, my patients who just randomly act and take steps that are not at all in keeping with their personal values or their best vision of themselves, often feel bad about the outcomes of their actions when things don't go well.

Having a plan in place, rather that reacting to what is in front of you, will give you the best chance of having a sense of control in college, living up to your personal standards, and being happy with the outcomes of your actions.

Step 4. <u>Practice the Power of the Word "No"</u>
College has many exciting experiences to participate in, but too much fun can be a distraction from your schoolwork and take you off your college path. You are going to need to learn to say "no" and focus on the most important reason you've gone to college—your future.

It is completely in your power to decide what is right for you, and just saying "no" can speak very clearly about your opinion. The word "no" is quite powerful. It often puts an end to the discussion because it says exactly how you feel.

There may be times in college that you get a feeling that you need to avoid a particular circumstance or get out of a situation that has already begun. First, trust your instincts. Next, be prepared by thinking of a few sentences you can say that will put an end to what is happening. Practice those sentences in advance of college so that they are clear in your mind and are ready to use if a difficult situation arises.

Pre-College Homework Part Two:
Detailed Questions to Think Through in Advance

<u>"What Kind of Woman Do You Want to Be?"</u>
Only you can answer the question about who you really are and where you see yourself going in life. I would encourage you to draw upon your personal values and to set your standards high as you answer the questions below.

- What is really important to you?
- What motivates you?
- What are your goals?
- What are your talents?
- Whom do you admire? Who are your role models?

Think about how you feel about the lifestyle issues below. When answering the questions, keep in mind the best vision you have for yourself as a woman:

1. Approach to Life: Spontaneous? Planner? Just wing it?
2. Eating Habits: Health food? Junk food? Something in between?
3. Physical Activity: Do you exercise? Just want to sit around? Both?
4. Study Habits: Do you want to continue to improve your study habits? Procrastinate? Study ahead? Put forth your best? Just get by?
5. Religion/Spirituality: Is spirituality or religion a part of your life? Will you leave it behind when you move away from home? Explore other religions or spirituality?
6. Sexuality: Will you wait to have sex? Are you already sexually active? Do you want a committed relationship before starting to have sex? Do you see sexuality as something casual? Is it OK to have sex with an acquaintance or a friend? Will you be monogamous? Will you choose to have multiple sexual partners? Do your religious beliefs conflict with your opinion about sexuality?
7. Alcohol Use: Will you drink alcohol? Do you feel you have to drink alcohol to "fit in" or have fun? Do you have other activities you can do instead of drinking? How will you ensure your safety?
8. Stress Management: Do you feel that stress is a problem? Do you thrive on stress? How do you reduce your stress?
9. Loneliness: How do you feel about moving away from home? Are you afraid to make new friends? What will you do to feel comfortable and "at home" in college?
10. Depression: Have you ever felt down? Have you had a hard time handling your emotions? How will you seek help if you feel depressed?

What Are Your Boundaries?

It's very important to identify what makes you comfortable and uncomfortable in different social situations before you go to college. Understanding your boundaries will help you stay safe, make decisions consistent with the woman you want to be, and develop healthy relationships.

1. What qualities are you looking for in a roommate?

2. Can your roommate use your stuff? Does she have to ask you?
3. If you want people over, do you have to ask your roommate? Is there advanced notice required or can people just show up?
4. Are there set study hours in your room? What if you want to study late at night?
5. Will you sneak alcohol into your dorm room? What if your roommate sneaks in alcohol? How will you handle it if your roommate is drunk frequently in your room?
6. How will you communicate to your roommate that she is bothering you? Text; leave a note; email; talk it out?
7. If you have a partner (boyfriend, girlfriend)... is it OK for the partner to visit at any time? Stay overnight? Do the same rules apply to your roommate's partner?
8. If you are lesbian, gay, bisexual or transgender, do you care if your roommate is of a different sexual orientation?
9. If you are straight, do you care if your roommate is lesbian, gay, bisexual or transgender?
10. How will you feel if your roommate is not of the same race, socioeconomic situation or religion?
11. Will you welcome people of a different race, religion, socioeconomic situation or sexual orientation into your life?

Understand What's Ahead in College & Make Your Plan

I find that most young women do not know what's ahead for them in college, and therefore haven't thought about how to handle things in a safe and healthy way. Understanding the many health and social issues you will face in college enables you to be prepared. BEFORE you move out on your own, review the following situations to think about how you can best take care of yourself. I have seen that advanced planning can lead to the healthiest outcomes. Hindsight is never the best strategy.

Your Health
- What you'll eat
- Vitamins you'll take
- How you will exercise
- What you'll do if you have problems with your period, infections, or feel run down or depressed
- How you will balance your schedule so you can get enough sleep

Your Safety
- How you feel about your sexuality
- What you'll do to protect yourself from STDs and unplanned pregnancy
- Steps you'll take for safe alcohol use
- Precautions you'll take to avoid sexual assault
- What you will do if you are offered someone else's prescription medications

Your Happiness
- What you will do to handle stress
- How you'll handle difficult situations with your roommate, new friends, and your professors
- Steps you will take to study and stay on top of your schoolwork
- How you can move forward after making a mistake
- What you'll do for a self-esteem boost
- What tools and apps you can use to stay on top of it all

Practice Sentences to Help You Say "No" in Difficult Situations

Based on my experience as a gynecologist, I have listed some sentences for you to use when facing a difficult situation in college. I have also included suggestions made by my patients. Ultimately, you should decide for yourself what makes you comfortable. The most important part is to practice a few sentences in advance of going to college so you feel confident that you know what to say if a difficult situation arises. Then review these occasionally.

- "No, I can't leave the party with you. I'm staying with my friends. Maybe we could meet up tomorrow after class."
- "No, I don't want any more alcohol. My stomach hurts."
- "No, I don't want to do shots. The last time I did, I threw up."
- "No, I'm not ready for sex."
- "No, I don't want to have sex. I just got my period, and it's really heavy. I need to go home."
- "Eww, what is that bump? I can't have sex with you because you have bumps down there."
- "No, I don't take drugs/snort coke/smoke pot. No!"
- "No, I don't want your prescription medication. I don't have (illness), and I have allergic reactions to most drugs."

- "No, I can't go out tonight because I have an exam, but let's meet up this weekend."
- "No, I can't do your homework for you because I have too much of my own. Maybe you can ask the professor for help."
- "No, I don't want to see the stolen test. I don't want to be accused of cheating."

Final Thoughts

Maybe you feel like you have all the answers to the Pre-College Homework and don't need any further clarification... if so, that's wonderful, and you should move forward in college. Perhaps, instead, this seems confusing because you haven't thought about these issues before, or you really don't know how you feel about these topics. No worries, I can help. We will cover everything in detail in the following chapters so you can understand what's ahead, give further thought to how YOU want to handle the health and social issues you will face, and feel confident as you forge ahead on your college path.

I want you to have a fabulous time in college, stay on track for your goals, and feel great about yourself as you navigate your way through some of the best years of your life. By getting YOU prepared with a solid sense of who you are, and an understanding of what college is all about, you will have the tools you need to be healthy and safe, and enjoy all the amazing college experiences ahead.

Be Healthy

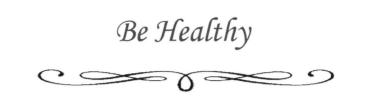

When I went to college, I gained a lot of weight. Not the "Freshman 15"...for me it was the Freshman 50! I don't have a single stretch mark from having three children, but I do have stretch marks from freshman year.

I lived in the only all-girls dorm on my college campus. We went to the cafeteria at 4:30 p.m. when many of the men's sports teams would go to eat. The athletes would eat a lot of food because they were obviously working out intensely as part of their athletic routine. I was not working out at all. I had never seen more food in one place as I did in the college cafeteria. There were 40 flavors of ice cream, and I tried every one.

There was one girl from my dorm who didn't gain any weight. I asked her one day what her "trick" was to avoid putting on the pounds. She said something that has stuck with me forever. She looked me in the eye and said, "I choose to be thin." Hmmm.....I found that sentence so annoying at the time. Her words were harsh, but they really got me thinking. I realized that I had no plan for how to eat and was just randomly approaching my life. I wanted to be healthier and felt motivated to make a change.

It took me all year to lose the weight, and I never put it back on except when I was pregnant. How I lost the weight was a combination of willpower and a clear nutrition and exercise plan. I went to see a registered dietitian who taught me about smart food choices. I didn't have to be perfect, but I needed to know what to eat the majority of the time. I thought of that girl from my dorm with the sassy comment every time I went for something that was not on my plan for healthy eating. I'd ask myself, "Is this worth the calories?" Further, I started to exercise by doing aerobics and riding my bike.

Now you know my story! I learned the hard way about the importance of a healthy lifestyle in my freshman year. By incorporating a balanced daily routine into my life during college, I have been able to maintain my health and weight during the following 25 years.

In addition to good nutrition and regular exercise, being healthy requires getting enough sleep, recognizing the symptoms of depression, and knowing when to go to the doctor for common medical problems. The following chapters will outline what you need to know.

Remember, no one is perfect and everyone makes mistakes. That's OK. The goal is to understand how you can take good care of yourself and to "choose to be healthy" when you move out on your own.

Chapter 2
Make Healthy Food Choices

When you go to college, it may be the first time in your life that you will have to figure out what to eat every day. Maybe you will go to the college cafeteria and eat whatever is there; or you'll go to the local fast-food restaurant and have your favorite burger, fries, and pop. Neither of these approaches is ideal and can lead to poor nutrition or obesity. I realize that it can be very difficult to know what to eat, especially when the college "food court" is providing almost any food you can imagine. What you eat matters, so learning how to eat with these guidelines now will help you avoid gaining weight in college and have the best health throughout your life.

Three Important Tips for Eating in College

There is abundant literature available about how to eat healthy on various websites, but it is often confusing and difficult to interpret the information. Frequently, the biggest challenge is applying the recommendations to your daily life.

To help you with this, I have three recommendations to keep in mind as you read through this chapter and then navigate your way through the college cafeteria.

1. Be an educated eater. It's important to know what you need to eat and what is in the foods you are eating. We are each unique, which is why one diet is not perfect for everyone. The following guidelines are a great start to healthy eating. As your activity levels change, make adjustments in your calorie and nutrient intake.

2. Eat more fruits and veggies. Pick a variety of different colorful fruits and vegetables as a low-calorie source of vitamins, minerals, fiber, and antioxidants.

3. Avoid processed foods when possible. Your body is designed to eat food that's closest to its natural state. While preservatives enable you to eat foods that are out of season, processed foods are loaded with sodium and chemical additives that do little to nourish your body.

We all need energy to live, breath, and keep our bodies moving. Energy is measured in calories, just as length is measured in feet and weight is measured in pounds. Every woman requires a different amount of energy based on her age, weight, and level of activity.

Food Guidelines for Freshman Year

The Dietary Guidelines for Americans were updated in 2015. The recommendations for an average **18-year-old woman** are:

1,800 to 2,400 calories per day

- 5-6 ½ ounces or 46 grams of protein (lean meats/beans)
- 1 ½-2 cups of fruit
- 2 ½-3 cups of veggies
- 6-8 oz. grains (to include 3-4 oz. of whole grains)
- 3 cups low-fat dairy
- Less than 10% of calories from saturated fat

See specific examples of what to eat in the "Healthy Foods List" at the end of this chapter.

Try to eat approximately 1,800 calories per day if you are a "non-active" college woman, meaning the main form of physical activity you do is casually walking to and from class every day.

If you are a "moderately physically active" woman, increase your intake to 2,000 calories daily. This would describe a woman who walks quickly through campus, bikes less than 10 mph or participates in water aerobics.

If you are a "very physically active" woman, increase your intake to 2,400 calories daily. This describes a woman who jogs, runs, plays basketball, does aerobics, or swims at a moderate to high speed.

If you are a competitive athlete or participate in an aggressive training program, the guidelines above do not apply to you. Please talk to the team nutritionist or school dietitian to get the specific caloric and dietary recommendations for you.

<u>Food Guidelines for Sophomore to Senior Year</u>
According to the 2015 Dietary Guidelines, once you are **19 years old and beyond**, your daily calorie and nutrition intake should be:
- "Non-active" women: 2,000 calories
- "Moderately physically active" women: 2,200 calories
- "Very physically active" women: 2,400 calories
- 5-6 ½ ounces or 46 grams of protein (lean meats/beans)
- 2 cups of fruit
- 2 ½-3 cups of veggies
- 6-8 oz. of grains (to include 3-4 oz. whole grains)
- 3 cups of low-fat dairy
- Less than 10% of calories from saturated fat

Understand What is In the Food You are Eating

Whenever possible, look on the food label with the nutrition facts to see how many calories and how much fat, sugar, sodium, and protein the product contains. This will help you become an educated eater.

What is a **high-calorie or low-calorie** food or drink?
According to the U.S. Food and Drug Administration:
- Food/drinks with 40 calories are considered low calorie.
- Food/drinks with 100 calories are considered moderate calorie.
- Food/drinks with greater than 250 calories are high calorie.

How much **fat** do I need?
Fat is a nutrient found in food, and it contains the most calories compared to other nutrients. It is important to not only choose healthy fats, but to eat an appropriate amount of fat in order to prevent weight gain and heart disease. See the Healthy Foods List at the end of this chapter for several examples of healthy fats to choose.

The daily saturated fat recommendation is listed as a percentage of daily calories. This calculation can be difficult, so you may prefer to think of it as a "certain amount of saturated fat to spend each day." Ask yourself how you want to spend it? This approach may help you skip fattening snacks.
- Look on the food label to see the number of grams of total and saturated fat in the food you are choosing.

- 1,800 daily calories: Limit total fat to 50-70 grams/day. Saturated fat should be limited to less than 20 grams/day.
- 2,400 daily calories: Total fat range limit is 53-93 grams/day. Saturated fat should be limited to less than 27 grams/day.
- The American Heart Association has a calculator for your daily fat and calorie needs. Their guidelines are a bit strict but it's an easy tool to use. Find it at myfatstranslator.com/

What **types of fats** should I avoid?

1. Saturated fats: solid animal fat, such as butter, margarine, baking grease (lard), and the fat around meat.
2. Trans fats (hydrogenated or partially hydrogenated oils): found in many snacks. The AHA recommends no more than 2 grams of trans fat daily. It's best to choose food with 0 grams of trans fat.

What is a **low-fat** food or drink?

A food or drink is defined as "low fat" when 30 percent or less of its calories are from fat. The best way to figure this out is to take a look at the label. For every 100 calories, if the food or drink has 3 grams or less of fat, it's considered low fat.

What is the most amount of **sugar** I should consume daily?

There are no specific recommended limitations for *natural sugar* found in fruit, vegetables, and milk. Follow the Food Guidelines on pg. 22-23 for the amount of fruit, veggies and dairy you need daily.

It is the *added sugar* in food and drinks that is unhealthy, adds calories, and should be limited. According to the AHA, the maximum added sugar women should consume daily is 100 calories, which is equivalent to 25 grams or 6 teaspoons.

Look on the food label to see how much sugar is in the food/drinks you consume. The *total sugar* on the label will include both natural and added sugars.

Look on the ingredients list to help you understand how much *added sugar* is in your food/drinks. If one of the first three ingredients listed is sugar or a sugar equivalent (dextrose, high fructose corn syrup, brown sugar, honey, cane juice, molasses, nectar), the product contains a high amount of added sugar.

<u>What is the recommended daily amount of **sodium** that
I should limit my diet to?</u>

- The 2015 Dietary Guidelines recommend to limit daily sodium to 2,300 mg. Greater amounts can cause high blood pressure.
- If you have diabetes, kidney disease, hypertension or a genetic predisposition for hypertension, the daily recommendation of sodium is 1,500 mg. It can be difficult to achieve this strict limit, so any reduction is beneficial.
- Your specific medical conditions may impact your individual sodium needs and should be discussed with your doctor.

At the time of this updated publication in 2016, the Dietary Guidelines listed for all nutrients are current. These guidelines are reviewed and updated every five years, so talk to your doctor about future changes.

Vitamins/Nutrients You Need

If you have a balanced diet, research shows that you can skip taking vitamins. However, many college students may not have a balanced diet and would benefit from supplements supplying the following nutrients:

- Calcium, 500-600 mg twice daily--builds strong bones and teeth.
- Vitamin D3, 600 IU daily--builds strong bones and may reduce some cancers. Many people, especially those with limited sun exposure, may benefit from additional vitamin D and should talk to their doctor.
- Omega-3 fatty acids, 1,100 mg daily--helps with brain power; heart health; skin and hair health; anti-inflammatory benefits.
- Vitamin A, 700 mg/day; Vitamin C, 65-75 mg/day; and Vitamin E, 15 mg/day-- antioxidants that support a healthy immune system, reduce inflammation, and improve healing.
- B-complex--for energy and metabolism.
- Zinc, 8-9 mg daily--supports a healthy immune system for wellness.
- Iron, 15-18 mg daily--maintains healthy blood to help avoid anemia.
- Magnesium, 300-360 mg daily--increases energy and helps avoid muscle aches; some literature on benefit for headaches.

If you are a competitive athlete, or participate in a training program, you will need additional vitamins and nutrients. Talk to the team nutritionist or a registered dietitian.

All Vitamins are Not Created Equal

My daughters are very active in sports and sometimes, like all teens on the run, do not have the healthiest of diets. I want them to have adequate vitamins, so I purchased a food-based "teen vitamin" from the local whole foods grocery store. Always look on the back of the vitamin bottle to be sure you're getting as healthy a vitamin as possible. If you have food sensitivities or intolerances, consider a vitamin brand that is free of artificial flavors, colors, and preservatives. If you have allergies, make sure the vitamin does not contain the item you are allergic to. For concerns about gluten, wheat, soy or fish, you may need to call the manufacturer. Look for the U.S. Pharmacopeia (USP) seal on supplement labels, which indicates that the company has chosen to follow higher quality standards to assure the product is as advertised.

Talk to Your Doctor before Taking Any Vitamin or Supplement

Your doctor will need to make sure the supplements/vitamins do not interfere with any other medications you may be taking and do not affect any medical conditions you may have.

Science Changes and So Do Vitamin Recommendations

The vitamin and nutrition information outlined above is based on the American Congress of Ob/Gyne's *Clinical Updates* on Nutrition from July 2014. Always review the most recent medical information with your doctor before starting any vitamins or supplements.

Follow the Directions on the Bottle

"More is not necessarily better" is definitely true when it comes to vitamins. It is important to carefully follow the directions on the bottle to avoid consuming too much of each vitamin, unless directed differently by your doctor.

Website to Review Supplements

Since the FDA does not regulate supplements, be wise and know what you are putting into your body. Many websites and vitamin stores will try to sell you something for an "added benefit," however the research does not support the claim. If you are considering taking any supplement, ask your doctor first. For further info, look on the USDA Food and Nutrition Information Center's website, http://fnic.nal.usda.gov/dietary-supplements.

Breakfast Suggestions

According to the Academy of Nutrition and Dietetics, eating breakfast leads to better performance, concentration, and problem-solving skills. Other research indicates it reduces hunger during the day, which may help women avoid gaining weight in college. Adding protein at breakfast has been shown in some studies to lead to greater satiety and less hunger later in the day.

Healthy breakfast choices

- Greek yogurt with fresh blueberries. Add flax seed for extra crunch and a healthy source of omega 3 fatty acids; add cinnamon to yogurt for sweetness without the calories; or blend these ingredients with frozen fruit for a homemade smoothie.
- Oatmeal with low-fat milk. Top with berries and mixed nuts.
- Scrambled eggs or an omelet, each is a great source of protein. Add cheese for calcium and extra protein; add veggies for vitamins and fiber.
- Breakfast cereals: Low-sugar, whole grain cereals are a good choice. If you don't like whole grain, pick a protein-enriched cereal for additional nutrition.
- Fresh fruit is loaded with vitamins; pair it with protein sources like eggs and cheese.
- Blend a green smoothie for a fast, healthy breakfast full of antioxidants and vitamins. Many websites have great green smoothie recipes to try. The basics include apples, cucumbers, spinach, ginger, celery, and limes. Some recipes add kale and parsley. See what you like best.
- Consider an instant breakfast drink packet for a fast start to your day. Look on the food label to compare brands and pick one that contains 10-20 grams of protein and has less than 20 grams of sugar. The No-Added-Sugar Carnation Instant Breakfast is a good choice.
- Grab a cheese stick when you're on the run.

- Make a homemade protein shake with powdered protein, Greek yogurt, and fresh fruits or veggies. There are several types of protein, however, whey protein is absorbed the best.
- If your only option is to stop at a fast-food restaurant, try to limit your choices to an egg burrito or egg sandwich that contain less than 20 grams of fat.
- Brew a cup of green or black tea, each loaded with antioxidants.
- Drink coffee with low-fat milk for a source of calcium.
- Try sugar-free iced coffee. It has 0 grams of sugar.
- Have a glass of orange or grapefruit juice for healthy vitamins.
- Drink a large glass of water each morning. Drinking water meets a hydration need, which once satisfied, eliminates a false hunger feeling.

Breakfast Food and Drinks to Avoid (or maybe just have on weekends)

- Sugary cereals
- Frosted tarts for the toaster, doughnuts, and sugary muffins
- Breakfast sandwiches with sausage, biscuits, and gravy that are greater than 20 grams of fat
- Deep-fried hash browns that have more than 20 grams of fat
- Coffee loaded with caramel, mocha, sugar, and whipped cream
- Pop
- Store-bought protein shakes and smoothies unless the labels indicate that they contain at least 20 grams of protein and less than 45 grams of carbohydrates. Store-bought protein shakes and smoothies may be a nutritional benefit or a caloric nightmare. Read the labels or get the nutritional info online. A meal replacement drink or smoothie with less than 15 grams of protein, more than 45 grams of carbohydrates, and 300 calories will not provide the best health benefit. Unless you are carb-loading for a sport event, skip these drinks.

Understand the Amount of Sugar in Your Breakfast Coffee Drink

One teaspoon of granulated sugar = 4 grams of sugar.
A coffee drink with 16 grams of sugar means that the drink contains four teaspoons of granulated sugar.

- Grande (16-ounce) unsweetened iced coffee: 0 grams of sugar
- Grande sweetened iced coffee: 20 grams (5 teaspoons) of sugar

- Grande low-fat latte: 18 grams (4 ½ teaspoons) of sugar
- Grande vanilla bean frappuccino, non-fat milk and no whipped cream: 67 grams (16 ¾ teaspoons) of sugar in one drink

Other Sugary Drinks

Pop: a 12-ounce can of pop contains about 10 teaspoons of sugar
Chai tea lattes: a medium cup contains about 10 teaspoons of sugar
Energy drinks: a small can contains about 5 ½ teaspoons of sugar
Sports drinks: a 20-ounce bottle contains about 8 teaspoons of sugar

Women who struggle with their weight are often drinking too many sweetened drinks. They don't realize how much the large amount of sugar they are consuming significantly affects their weight.

As a reminder, the maximum amount of added sugar that a woman should consume per day is 6 teaspoons, 25 grams or 100 calories. There are many foods and drinks that contain added sugar, so try to avoid the daily pop, juice smoothies, and coffee drinks made with caramel, mocha, and whipped cream. Instead, choose these drinks for a special treat.

How Much Water Should You Drink?

Sixty percent of our body weight comes from water. Insufficient water intake can lead to fatigue and dehydration. Water is calorie-free, readily available, inexpensive, and can give you more energy. Pop, on the other hand, is loaded with sugar and sodium, and can lead to tooth decay, dehydration, and obesity. So drink water and skip the pop.

The Institute of Medicine recommends:
- Women need to drink 9 cups of total liquids per day.
- Water should be the beverage of choice.

Mayo Clinic recommends:
- Modify water intake based on amount of physical activity, college climate, and individual health status.
- Aerobic activity that leads to sweating requires an extra 1½ to 2½ cups of water per day.

- Intense aerobic activity requires more than just water. It's better to drink a sports drink with electrolytes (such as Gatorade or Powerade) when engaging in intense physical activity.
- Increase water intake if you go to college in a hot climate or located at an altitude higher than 8,200 feet.

Helpful App

Add an app to your smartphone to help you remember to drink enough water. One app my patients like is Watermind Me. You can track your water intake and set reminders.

Helpful Hint

When in doubt, look at your urine. If it is dark like tea, you are not drinking enough water. Urine should be clear or have a faint yellow color similar to lemonade.

Dorm Room Basics

There are many books you can buy to tell you what you should be bringing to college with you. My dorm list is based on getting enough nutrition while in school and helping you avoid grabbing something unhealthy while you're on the go. **I've listed many items below, but don't be overwhelmed because you don't have to buy everything on the list.** I want you to have some options, so choose what fits your needs.

- Buy a compact, inexpensive **blender or "Magic Bullet"** to have in your room to make a quick smoothie for breakfast, or anytime you are hungry, rather than grabbing a doughnut on the go.
- Rent or purchase a **refrigerator with a small freezer**.
- Bring a few **glass storage containers** and **small freezer bags** for freezing.
- In your fridge, keep **Greek yogurt** for its protein and probiotic benefits; store **ground flax seed** in a sealed container for a great source of fiber and omega 3 fatty acids, and possible benefit to reduce breast and colon cancers; have a few **low-fat cheese sticks** on hand for a snack on the go.
- In your freezer, keep **frozen fruit** for a healthy vitamin boost in your smoothies or as a snack on their own. You can purchase organic frozen blueberries and strawberries from the grocery

store. You can also freeze your own peeled bananas, grapes, pineapples, and berries in a glass container.

- If you like to make green smoothies, you can freeze **green leafy veggies** like spinach and kale in small freezer bags; or purchase these greens already frozen.
- Store some **unsalted mixed nuts** in a cool dry place. Snacking on nuts keeps your cholesterol levels in a healthy range and maintains heart health.
- Keep some **fresh fruit,** such as bananas, oranges, blueberries or apples in your room for a healthy snack.
- If you have a kitchen in your dorm, store **brown rice** for its antioxidant benefit, vitamins and fiber. Keep several types of **beans** on hand to reduce inflammation, add fiber, and provide antioxidant benefits. Store **whole oats**, full of vitamins and fiber, to make a healthy oatmeal breakfast or bake an oatmeal cookie treat.
- Buy **black and green tea** for the antioxidant benefits, heart health, and to reduce the risk of colon and pancreatic cancer.
- Store ground **cinnamon** to add to your coffee, cereal, or sprinkle on fruit for sweetness without the calories. Cinnamon is an antioxidant and stabilizes blood sugar.
- **Ginger,** stored fresh or in ground form, has anti-inflammatory benefits and reduces nausea if you are not feeling well. It can be added to tea, cookies, or smoothies. **Turmeric**, from the ginger family, helps fight inflammation and reduces risk of some cancers. Store ginger and turmeric, along with any **vitamins** you may be taking, in a cool dark place.
- **Fat-free, low-sugar salad dressing**, such as Walden Farms, can be stored in your refrigerator to use on a take-out salad or as dip for veggies. Or better yet, buy plain yogurt and add dried salad seasoning for a homemade dip or dressing.

Healthy Food List

College cafeterias have many food choices, including options that are not very healthy. A good rule of thumb is to choose food from the following food list at least 80 percent of the time for healthy eating in college. You can still enjoy other things, but not every day.

Keep the following food list handy so it can be a quick reference when you navigate through the cafeteria. Stick to the recommended amount of each type of nutrient to avoid overeating.

Protein: Lean Meat/Beans

College-age women need 5-6 ½ ounces or 46 grams of protein daily.
Typically one ounce = seven grams of protein

(The additional grams of protein needed to meet the daily requirements can be met with protein from dairy and, to a lesser degree, veggies and grains.)

- One slice of turkey for a sandwich (1/8 inch-thick) = one ounce
- One slice of low-sodium deli ham (1/8 inch-thick)   = one ounce
- One tablespoon peanut butter (thumb-sized scoop) = one ounce
- One tablespoon almond butter (thumb-sized scoop)= one ounce
- One egg   = one ounce
- 12 almonds, 24 pistachios or seven walnut halves   = one ounce
- Two tablespoons humus (two thumb-sized scoops) = one ounce
- ¼ cup cooked beans (black, pinto, kidney, white)   = one ounce
- ¼ cup cooked peas (chickpeas, lentils, split peas)   = one ounce
- ¼ cup tofu   = one ounce
- One falafel patty   = one ounce
- ¼ cup roasted soybeans   = one ounce
- ½ cup Quinoa (gluten free, high fiber)   = one ounce

One ounce is about the size of a ping-pong ball.

- ¼ cup Greek yogurt   = two ounces
- Three egg whites   = two ounces
- One soy or bean burger patty   = two ounces
- One cup lentil or bean or split pea soup = two ounces

- One small lean hamburger   = three ounces
- One small chicken breast half   = three ounces
- One small piece of trout   = three ounces
- One small steak (round or filet) = 3-4 ounces
- One can of tuna, drained   = 3-4 ounces
- One piece of salmon filet   = 4-6 ounces

Three ounces is about the size of a deck of cards.

Fruits

18-year-old women need 1½-2 cups of fruit daily.
19 to 24-year-old women need 2 cups of fruit daily.
Fruits are full of vitamins, minerals, antioxidants and fiber.

- Cranberries
- Raspberries
- Tomatoes (medium size)
- Blackberries
- Strawberries
- Bananas (medium size)
- Blueberries
- Red or green grapes
- Oranges
- Cherries
- Apples (medium size)
- Mangos

One cup is about the size of your fist.

Veggies

College-age women need 2 ½-3 cups of vegetables daily.

Anytime you are hungry, snack on veggies because they are loaded with nutrition and generally do not cause women to gain weight.

- Green leafy veggies (lettuces)
- Cucumbers
- Broccoli
- Brussel sprouts
- Yellow, orange, and red peppers
- Cauliflower
- Green beans
- Carrots
- Beets
- Mushrooms
- Chili peppers

One cup is about the size of your fist.

Grains
College-age women need 6-8 ounces of grains daily.
At least 3-4 ounces should be whole grains.

Whenever possible, choose whole grains instead of white breads and pastas for the beneficial fiber, iron and B vitamins.

- One slice of sandwich bread
  (Wheat, sourdough or whole grain)   = one ounce
- One small slice of French bread   = one ounce
- Seven square or round saltines or snack crackers = one ounce
- Five whole wheat crackers or two rye crisps   = one ounce
- One mini-bagel or half of an English muffin   = one ounce
- One small (golf-ball size) muffin   = one ounce
- ½ cup cooked oatmeal (whole oats cereal)   = one ounce
- One buttermilk pancake (4 ½-inch diameter)   = one ounce
- Three cups popped popcorn   = one ounce
- ½ cup cooked rice
  (Brown, wild or white enriched)   = one ounce
- ½ cup Quinoa, couscous or barley   = one ounce
- One small 6-inch corn tortilla   = one ounce

- One mini bag of microwave low-fat popcorn   = two ounces
- One cup cooked pasta (whole wheat)   = two ounces

- One large bagel   = four ounces
- One large 12-inch flour tortilla   = four ounces

Low-Fat Dairy
College-age women need 3 cups of low-fat dairy daily.

- Low-fat yogurt   4-ounce snack size   = ½ cup
- Natural cheese:
  (Cheddar, Mozzarella or Swiss) one slice (1 ½ oz.) = ½ cup
- Cottage cheese   one-cup container   = ½ cup

- Low-fat milk   one cup   = one cup
- Soy milk   one cup   = one cup

Healthy Fats

Limit total fat to 25-35 percent of daily calories.
Limit saturated fat to 10 percent of daily calories.
Limit TOTAL FAT to 44-93 grams per day, depending on your calories, with a focus on **healthy fats**. Total fat includes fat you add to your meal (added fat), plus fat found in food (hidden fat). **Limit intake of SATURATED FAT to less than 20-27 grams per day**, depending on your calories. The goal for the new 2015 guidelines is to minimize saturated fats. Look on the food label for the *Total fat* and *Saturated fat* grams to monitor your fat intake and be healthy.
Three to five servings of ADDED FAT per day is sufficient.
This equals 15-25 grams of added fat daily.

Examples of Healthy Added Fats

Avocado (mashed)	1/8 of an avocado or 2 Tbsp.	= 1 serving
Olive oil	1 teaspoon	= 1 serving
Peanut oil	1 teaspoon	= 1 serving

One serving is approximately = 5 grams of added fat
1 tablespoon (Tbsp.) is the size of your thumb
1 teaspoon (tsp.) is the size of your thumbnail

Food with Healthy Hidden Fats

Nuts	4-6 nuts	= 5 grams
Salmon	3 ounces (size of deck of cards)	= 15 grams
Flaxseed	1½ Tbsp. (ground)	= 5 grams

Helpful Apps and Websites

I find it easiest to calculate the percentage of calories, protein, carbs, and fats using my Fitbit, but there are many apps and websites to help you understand what you are eating and to maintain your health. Some examples are My Fitness Pal app, SparkPeople.com, and SuperTracker on Choosemyplate.gov.

Helpful Tip

When in doubt about what or how much to eat, use the "plate method." Fill half your plate with colorful vegetables; add lean meat or another protein food to one-quarter of the plate; then fill the remaining quarter of your plate with a whole grain. If you're still hungry, have a cup of low-fat milk or yogurt and a piece of fruit.

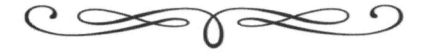

*"Learning to eat well is a
lifelong occupation.
Start now."*

*-Susan Rizzo, RD, LDN, CDE
Registered Dietitian*

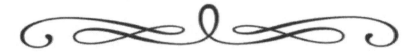

Chapter 3
Tips to Avoid Gaining Weight in College

Top Reasons Why Women Gain Weight in College
1. Eating too much food.
2. Eating meals that contain too much *added* sugar.
3. Drinking too much fruit juice, pop, and energy/sports drinks.
4. "Stress Eating."
5. Eating too many snacks between meals.
6. Eating food late at night.
7. Eating too much fast food.
8. Drinking too much alcohol.
9. No longer doing the exercise previously done in high school.
10. "Hanging out" a lot and not being active.

What is Your Healthy Target Weight Range?

- There is no perfect weight for your body. In fact, there is a range of weight that is considered healthy for every woman. The Body Mass Index is a helpful guide for you to identify a target weight range to maintain throughout your life. It's not a perfect measure but a very good reference for most women.
- The healthy goal for most women is a BMI between 18.5 and 24. Most BMI charts start with a BMI of 19.
- To calculate your BMI, look at the BMI Chart on the next page and find your height. Then move across the chart to the right to find what weight is listed in the column for a BMI of 19. This is the lowest healthy weight for your height. Now move across the chart to the right to find a BMI of 24. This would be the highest healthy weight for your height. Try to keep your weight in this ideal weight range for your health.
- A BMI of 25 is considered overweight, and a BMI of 30 is considered obese. A BMI less than 18.5 is considered underweight. Do your best to maintain a BMI of 18.5-24.

BMI Chart

BMI	19	20	21	22	23	24	25	26	27	28	29	30	31	32	33	34
Height							Weight in Pounds									
4'10	91	96	100	105	110	115	119	124	129	134	138	143	148	153	158	162
4'11	94	98	104	109	114	119	124	128	133	138	143	148	153	158	163	168
5'	97	102	107	112	118	123	128	133	138	143	148	153	158	163	168	174
5'1	100	106	111	116	122	127	132	137	143	148	153	158	164	169	174	180
5'2	104	109	115	120	126	131	136	142	147	153	158	164	168	175	180	186
5'3	107	113	118	124	130	135	141	146	152	158	163	169	175	180	186	191
5'4	110	116	122	128	134	140	145	151	157	163	169	174	180	186	192	197
5'5	114	120	126	132	138	144	150	156	162	168	174	180	186	192	198	204
5'6	118	124	130	136	142	148	155	161	167	173	179	186	192	198	204	210
5'7	121	127	134	140	146	153	159	166	172	178	185	191	198	204	211	217
5'8	125	131	138	144	151	158	164	171	177	184	190	197	203	210	216	223
5'9	128	135	142	149	155	162	169	176	182	189	196	203	209	216	223	230
5'10	132	139	146	153	160	167	174	181	188	195	202	209	216	222	229	236
5'11	136	143	150	157	165	172	179	186	193	200	208	215	222	229	236	243
6'	140	147	154	162	169	177	184	191	199	206	213	221	228	235	242	250
6'1	144	151	159	166	174	182	189	197	204	212	219	237	235	242	250	257
6'2	148	155	163	171	179	186	194	202	210	218	225	233	241	249	256	264

If your height or weight is outside this chart, refer to the National Institutes of Health website, www.nih.gov for information

Online BMI Calculator

There are many online BMI calculators, such as offered by Mayo Clinic, http://www.mayoclinic.org/bmi-calculator/itt-20084938

Sugar and Your Weight

Added sugar in food and drinks is thought to be associated with the high rate of obesity in the United States. As stated above, obesity is a BMI of 30. Too much sugar is linked to:

- Weight gain: Sugar adds a lot of calories to food and drinks.
- Poor nutrition: This occurs when sugary food is eaten instead of more nutritious food.
- An increased triglyceride level (storage form of sugar and fat): builds up in your blood vessels and leads to heart disease.
- Tooth decay: Sugar feeds the oral bacteria, which erode the enamel and cause cavities.

AHA Recommendations for Daily Added Sugar

As discussed in Chapter 2, women should not consume more than 100 calories per day from added sugar. That equates to six teaspoons, or 25 grams, of added sugar daily.

Strategy for Healthy Eating to Avoid Gaining Weight

1. **Have a clear nutrition plan in place, an exercise routine to follow, and the willpower to stick to your plans.** It may sound tough, but this approach gets easier with time and can work for most college women.
2. **Understand the importance of portion control.** You can gain weight even by eating healthy food if you're eating too much of it. See the Healthy Food List for recommended amounts to eat.
3. **Take your time eating and stop when you feel satisfied.** It takes 20 minutes for the stomach to tell the brain that it is full. If you eat on the run, you may overeat and not feel full until 15 minutes later. Instead, take your time while eating so you will get a feeling of fullness during the meal and not eat so much.
4. **Add some apps (listed on the next page) to your smartphone to help you keep track of your food intake, activities, and calories.** It has been shown that people who monitor and record their food intake lose more weight when needed.
5. Look at the **"Healthy Food List," the "Food/Drinks to Minimize," and the "Food/Drinks to Avoid" lists** on the next few pages. Take a picture of the lists with your phone so you can reference them regularly. **Review the "Food Guidelines"** for your age on pages 22-23 of Chapter 2.
6. **Find out what the cafeteria will be serving each day of the week.** Most colleges list the exact meals being served in the cafeteria each day on the college website in the "meals" section.
7. **Compare** your "Healthy Foods List" to the meals that the cafeteria will be serving to choose what you will eat each day. Use the "Food Guidelines" to help you decide upon your meal.
8. *THIS IS THE MOST IMPORTANT STEP:* **Plan in advance what you'll be eating each day BEFORE you go into the cafeteria, and then stick to the plan**. Go straight to the food that you planned to eat, and then walk away from the rest of the food choices. Eat only that food, and then leave the cafeteria.
9. If you're still hungry when done with your plate, go back for seconds of veggies or salad (watch the butter & salad dressing).
10. If it's a special event and you really want to enjoy a certain food, then you should go for it. Everyone should enjoy a dessert, pizza, a big bowl of pasta or a cheeseburger once in a while. These choices are fine if enjoyed occasionally.

Apps to Help You Avoid Gaining Weight in College

- **MyFitnessPal:** www.myfitnesspal.com/apps
  This is a great app to help you track your calories and exercise. It also has information about the nutrients in the food offered in different restaurants so you will know what you are consuming before you eat out. The nutrition database is also quite helpful.
- **MapMyWalk:** www.mapmywalk.com
- **MapMyRun:** www.mapmyrun.com
- **MapMyRide:** www.mapmyride.com
  These three apps are great for exercise monitoring, tracking how far you traveled, how fast, and how long you worked out. They download the information onto your computer so you can keep track of it and compare workouts over time.

Devices to Help You Stay Healthy and Fit

- **Fitbit:** www.fitbit.com/product
  This easy-to-use device is great to track your exercise; how many steps taken, stairs climbed, active minutes, and calories burned. Log into the Fitbit website to input the exact food you've eaten. The website will automatically calculate the calories you've consumed and indicate how many more you can have that day. It also calculates the protein, carbs, and percentage of fat you've consumed daily.
- **Mi-Pulse:** www. mi-pulse.com
  This is a brand new device coming to market in 2016. It is a revolutionary sports bra that includes an integrated heart rate monitor for accurate calorie counting and zone training without the hassle of a heart rate strap. It works using:
  - iPhones or Android-based smartphones
  - Leading sports watches
  - Various bike computers
  - Gym equipment that supports Polar

Helpful Websites

- **SparkPeople.com** provides a food tracker as well as exercise and motivation tips
- **SuperTracker** (from the USDA) tracks food intake; the site has additional tools to help with healthy eating
  http://www.choosemyplate.gov/supertracker-tools.html

Healthy Food List

The Healthy Food List is at the end of the last chapter, "Make Healthy Food Choices," and is based on the 2015 Dietary Guidelines. This list will help you understand what and how much of each type of food you should eat. Take a picture of the list on pages 32-35 and keep it handy for navigating the cafeteria.

Food/Drinks to Minimize

The following items contain a high amount of sugar and can easily increase your weight in college if you consume them too often or too much.
- Fruit juice (choose 100% juice, and limit it to 6 ounces per day)
- Sports drinks (may be indicated for athletes working out for more than four hours; otherwise water is best)
- Sweetened milk
- White bread, white pasta, white rice
- Cereal bars/granola (unless whole grain; look for bars with protein content greater than 7 grams)
- Flavored instant oatmeal (instead, choose unflavored oatmeal packs and add fresh fruit)
- Fruit cups in syrup/sweetened apple sauce cups
- Most salad dressings (they contain sugar, sodium and fat; limit dressing to 1-2 tablespoons.) (1 Tbsp. is the size of your thumb)
- Ketchup (limit to 1 Tbsp.)
- Pizza

Food/Drinks to Avoid

The following products should be routinely avoided because they contain high amounts of added sugar and little to no nutritional value. If you just love a particular item on this list, then have it when you want a special treat. Consuming any of these foods or drinks too frequently is unhealthy and can make you gain weight.
- Any food or drink that lists the first three ingredients as high fructose corn syrup, cane syrup, evaporated cane juice, malt syrup, molasses, brown rice syrup, added sugar or nectars
- Coffee with mocha, caramel, whipped cream or added syrup

- Pop
- Alcohol
- Sweetened iced tea
- Instant cocoa
- Fruit punch/fruit-flavored drinks
- Sugar-sweetened or frosted cereals
- Breakfast tarts
- Pudding/cookies/cake/candy

Things to Think About

- The abundance of available food is a big problem in college. It's great to have so many choices, but if you try to eat it all, you will gain weight. You need to have self-control.
- Eating more than one portion size of food can double the calories.
- The average American consumes more than 22 teaspoons of added sugar daily. You need to limit your intake of added sugar to six teaspoons, or 25 grams, per day.
- Take a look at the ingredients of what you consume.
- Regular pop usually contains high fructose corn syrup, while diet pop uses sugar substitutes for sweetness, which have no calories. As a rule of thumb, try to skip the pop and drink plenty of water.
- Put your snacks into a small bowl. Do not eat out of the large bag. Just 13-16 potato chips contain 155 calories and 10.62 grams of fat. If you sit with the bag, odds have it you'll consume even more, which leads to weight gain. Instead, pick a snack-size bag.
- Most salad dressings contain a lot of fat and added sugar. Try a brand, such as Walden Farms, that is free of fat and added sugar. Limit your intake to 1 Tbsp. (size of your thumb) because the sodium content in fat-free/sugar-free dressings can be high.
- Be aware that while the natural sugar in fruit is healthier than added sugars, it may add a lot of calories if you overdo it. Vegetables are always a good choice because they are lower in calories and also provide loads of vitamins and minerals. If you find you are not eating at least five servings of vegetables and fruits a day, you may want to consider a multivitamin to provide the nutrients you may be lacking.

- The average drive-thru cheeseburger and medium fries contains between 27 and 42 grams of fat and 630-860 calories—and that doesn't include the pop. The weight adds up when fast food becomes a daily habit.
- Students often forget about the empty calories and high-calorie ingredients in alcohol that can lead to weight gain.
- Each regular beer contains 100-180 calories and high carbohydrates; light beers have lower calories (60-99 calories) and fewer carbohydrates; either choice can make you gain weight if you consume too many.
- One ready-to-drink raspberry vodka drink contains 250 calories and 40 grams of carbohydrates. This type of beverage is considered a high-calorie drink with a high sugar load, which will lead to weight gain. The same applies to wine coolers and other mixed drinks.
- Beware of the term "Superfood." The media uses this word to describe a food that has supposed better nutrition compared to other foods and may help to minimize weight gain. There is not enough scientific evidence yet to tell people to focus their diet on any specific food because it is "super." In order to have a healthy, balanced diet, it is important to eat a variety of nutritious food. Science has not yet found one food that gives us all the nutrition we need.

Late-Night Eating

Friends may tempt you to go out for a pizza or burger at 2:00 a.m. after a party. This is a sure way to gain weight in college. The research has shown that eating at night is not the problem, but it is the extra calories consumed that lead to weight gain.

Oftentimes, students eat their usual calorie intake during the day, then add calories by drinking alcohol, followed by late-night binge eating. Those excess calories in the alcohol and late-night food, stored as fat, really add up and cause weight gain.

I'd encourage you to enjoy the social aspects of college, but minimize the alcohol and late-night eating. If you plan to go out at night, pay attention to the calories and sugar you consume throughout the day to avoid extra calories and to help you maintain a healthy weight.

Be aware that eating healthy and avoiding gaining weight does not equal not eating. You need to eat for a healthy body and mind, and finding balance in your nutrition should be your goal. You need nutrients to maintain weight, as well as lose weight in a healthy way. Eating disorders can develop as some women have difficulty with their body image and eating habits.

- Anorexia: Women suffering from this eating disorder have a distorted perception of how they look and truly believe they are "fat" when in reality, they are exceedingly thin. Their intense fear of gaining weight leads to an extreme self-restriction of food. In addition, it can lead to vomiting, excessive exercise, and use of laxatives, diet pills, and enemas. This disorder originates from difficulty coping with emotional problems and stress, which leads these women to associate their self-worth with being thin. This dangerous condition can lead to malnutrition and death. Counseling and diet education are important parts of healing.

- Bulimia: This eating disorder is also a result of trying to cope with emotional problems and stress, and can lead to malnutrition and death. Women with bulimia have a distorted body perception and take extreme measures to avoid gaining weight, such as purging/vomiting meals and taking laxatives. Despite the purging, women with bulimia are often normal weight or overweight. Counseling and diet education are important parts of healing.

If you find someone struggling or fear you have an eating disorder: Talk to the school health service or nutritionist, or call the National Eating Disorders Association hotline at 1-800-931-2237. To chat online, go to www.nationaleatingdisorders.org/find-help-support.

For further questions about how to maintain a healthy weight and avoid gaining weight in college, these are helpful websites: Heart.org, MyPlate.Gov, MayoClinic.org, and Eatright.org

Chapter 4
Exercise 101

After gaining 50 pounds my freshman year, I realized that I needed to find some exercise to do that was enjoyable. I started to ride my bike every day, which allowed me to get around campus easily, see all the surrounding areas of Boston, and get plenty of exercise - I loved it! In addition, I joined an aerobics class that met in my college gym four days a week. During the class, I met some nice friends who had common values of health and exercise. So instead of going out to a party at night after studying, we would meet to workout. After a few months of my new daily routine, I looked forward to the exercise and felt more energetic and happier overall.

Exercise pushes your body to release hormones called endorphins, which actually help you fight stress and make you feel good. So, in addition to the physical benefits from exercise, the emotional benefits you will receive from stress reduction will be very valuable.

Make Exercise Part of Your College Life

- **Have fun**. Figure out what activities are most enjoyable for you and will get your body moving. Put down the cell phone and join a volleyball club, make a goal to run a 5-kilometer race or sign up for an intramural team.

- **Make friends with similar values and healthy lifestyles**. Rather than choosing friends who only like to go to parties and drink alcohol for fun, find people who like to be physically active for enjoyment. Skip the bars and instead play tennis, hike across campus, join a dance class or workout together at the college gym for fun and a healthy friendship for many years.

- **Make it a priority**. Look at your college schedule to see how you can consistently add exercise to your daily college routine. Put it on your calendar and make it happen.

- **Be purposeful**. Aerobic physical activity should last at least 10 minutes at a time, spread throughout the week.

What Exercise Should You Do?

The first step is to put your shoes on and get moving. The recommendations below are a great guide; you only need 2 ½ hours of exercise per week to be healthy. Even more effort would be helpful. Start slowly and build up. Don't quit. Just keep trying.

The American Heart Association (AHA) Recommendations for Exercise

- 30 minutes of Moderate Intensity Aerobic Exercise* five days per week

  OR

- 45 minutes of Vigorous Intensity Aerobic Exercise** three days per week, PLUS Moderate- to High-Intensity Muscle-Strengthening Exercises*** two days per week

The U.S. Department of Health and Human Services Recommendations for Exercise

- 2 ½ hours/week of Moderate-Intensity Aerobic Exercise*

  OR

- 1 ¼ hours/week of Vigorous-Intensity Aerobic Exercise**

  OR

- A combination of both Moderate- and Vigorous-Intensity Aerobic Exercise for two hours/week

*Examples of Moderate-Intensity Aerobic Exercise
  o Walking 4 mph
  o Bicycling less than 10 mph
  o Water aerobics
  o Doubles tennis
  o Golf
  o Dancing

**Examples of Vigorous-Intensity Aerobic Exercise
- o Brisk walking 5 mph
- o Jogging 6 mph
- o Running 7 mph
- o Bicycling greater than 10 mph
- o Swimming laps
- o Singles tennis
- o Aerobics class
- o Basketball
- o Cross country skiing

***Examples of Moderate- to High-Intensity Muscle-Strengthening Exercise
- o Resistance training with bands
- o Weight training/lifting weights
- o Push-ups
- o Pull-ups
- o Sit-ups
- o Carrying heavy loads
- o Using the major muscle groups of the body including arms, shoulders, back, chest, abdomen, hips, and legs
- o Stop when it becomes difficult to do without help.

These same guidelines are recommended for women with disabilities. If these are not possible, adults with disabilities should be as physically active as their abilities allow.

Helpful App: RunKeeper: tracks and displays the paths you've taken as you walk, jog, bike or run. You can then compare distances you've traveled over time.

The next chapter will outline two different exercise routines that were designed for college women based on the recommended guidelines listed above. Try both step-by-step exercise routines in your dorm or at the gym to help you to be healthy and fit and feel great in college.

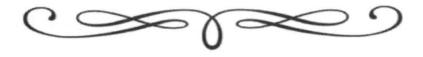

"You made it to college, which means you're a motivated person. Apply that same effort into exercise."

-Amy Winter
Fitness Expert

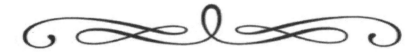

Chapter 5
Step-By-Step Exercise Routines In Your Dorm and At the Gym

Exercise is a very important part of being healthy, and the habits you make now will most likely stay with you for the rest of your life. If exercise is already part of your routine, then good for you! Keep it going! If you do not participate in some form of regular exercise, now's the time to get started! Maybe you just need some help because you don't really know what to do or where to begin--this chapter is a great place to start.

- The key to exercising in college is to schedule time for it into your day. Look at working out like attending a class--you need to be there, no excuses. Put your exercise plan into your cell phone calendar or assignment notebook so it's in front of you every day. Remember that any time you can devote to moving is better than none, so if you can only spare a few minutes, do it!
- Ideally, you should try to exercise for 30-60 minutes most days of the week.
- Change up your exercise plan every day so you don't get bored, and your body does not get accustomed to the program.
- Alternate between cardiovascular exercise (such as walking, running on a treadmill or riding a bike) and strength training. You should also do a combination of the two. Think about combining moves to get more out of your time.
- Be creative and figure out what works for you. If you have a test you need to study for, grab your book and find a machine like a stationary bike or elliptical where you can study and exercise at the same time. If you have extra time, try to do more.
- If you plan to go running, make sure you are in a safe area and never run alone at night.

Following are the "how to's" for college exercise. Check out the "Dorm Room or Apartment Workout" if you prefer privacy during exercise or the convenience of not leaving home. If you prefer to push yourself harder, try the "College Gym Workout" designed for the college rec-plex. To take the mystery out of what exercise to do each day, see the "One-Month Workout Schedule."

You can use these exercise routines as a guide or create your own. Try to change your plan at least every four weeks to keep it enjoyable. Making exercise fun and a part of your daily routine will help you develop a healthy lifestyle for the rest of your life.

Dorm Room or Apartment Workout

First, warm up for five to eight minutes:
  a. Jog in place
  b. Move side to side
  c. Squat and stand
  d. Reach overhead

Anything that gets your blood flowing and your body prepared for exercise will work.

Now do 10-15 repetitions of each of the following exercises:

- Push-ups (can be done on your knees or toes; straight back)

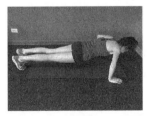

- Burpees (squat, stretch to a push-up, pull legs back in, then stand or jump to a standing position)

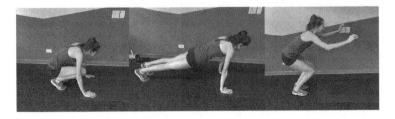

- Squats (your knees should be behind your toes and at a 45-degree angle; keep your back straight and shoulder blades pulled together)

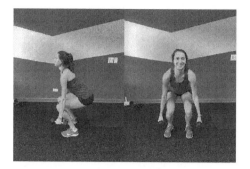

- Lunge right leg in front (back straight; front knee to 90 degrees; keep your front heel lined up with your back foot)

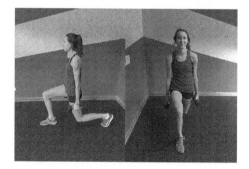

- Lunge left leg in front (pull your belly in to build your core and help you keep your balance)

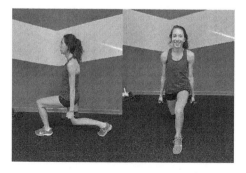

- Squat jumps (arms swing overhead when you jump; an easier option is to squat, then stand, without jumping)

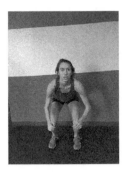

- Lunge jumps (try to keep your feet lined up; a less intense option is to step forward and back into a lunge rather than jumping)

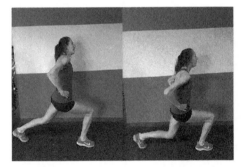

- Tricep dips (do this exercise on the edge of your bed; if this move is too difficult at first, try moving your feet closer to the bed)

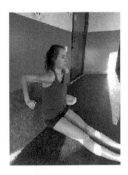

- Speed skate (place your foot back and tap while swinging your arms; jump into the pose; continue for 1 minute)

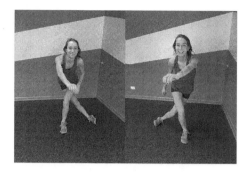

- Side plank with hip drops (stay on your elbow as you drop your hip down to the floor and back up; an easier option is to bend your lower leg and take some of the pressure off your arm)

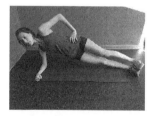

- Plank (relax your hands and look at the floor to keep your spine straight and take pressure off your neck; belly pulled in; shoulder blades pulled together; try to hold the position for 30 seconds to 1 minute)

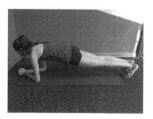

- Supine leg drops (alternate legs to the floor; hands beneath lower back, if support needed; bent knees are easier, if needed)

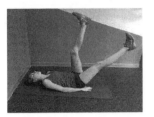

- Reverse curls (legs straight; do not swing your legs; lift hips off the ground while pushing your heels toward the ceiling)

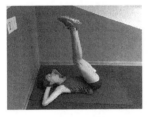

- Seated bicycling (kick back and forth; twisting torso)

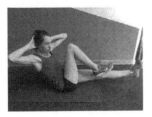

- One-leg balancing squat (pull belly in for balance; alternate legs)

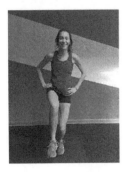

- 1-minute jumping jacks (touch the floor in between reps)
- Cool down by running or jogging in place for 3-4 minutes.

Do the above series two or three times if time allows.

The Benefit of Adding Hand Weights to Your Workout

1. The next time you do the "Dorm Room Workout," add 5- or 7-pound hand weights for greater toning, improved balance, and added strength.
2. It is better to do more repetitions with a lower weight than to injure yourself by lifting too much weight.

60-Minute College Gym Workout

If there is a student gym available on your college campus, you can increase the intensity and variety of your daily exercise routine.

Helpful equipment includes:
- Cardio machine
- Stability ball
- Resistance band
- 5- to 10-pound hand weights
- Medicine ball
- A step of some kind
- Cable machine

This workout includes high-intensity interval training as well as strength training. This approach will get your heart rate up to burn calories, improve fitness, and tone your body at the same time.

Caution: If you have any pain or injuries, wait to heal before you do this exercise routine. Prior to any fitness program, get your physician's approval.

Step-By-Step 60-Minute College Gym Workout

For pictures and additional descriptions for this workout, go to www.fteamtraining.com, click on "More" and then click on "*The Gyne's Guide 60 Minute College Gym Workout.*"

Start with a 5- to 10-minute warm-up such as jogging or use the elliptical machine to get your blood flowing and warm up your muscles.

Do 15 repetitions of the following movements:
- Push-ups
- Burpees
- Chest press on stability ball (put Pilates ball between your knees for added intensity)
- Weighted hip drops on stability ball
- Squats with dumbbells (start with a low weight and build up over time to avoid injury)
- Side lunge with biceps curl; alternate with the opposite side; do 15 repetitions on each side
- Jumping jacks with medicine ball (1 minute); touch the floor with the ball in between repetitions for added intensity
- Squat jumps (touch the floor in between) (1 minute)
- Speed skate with medicine ball (1 minute)
- One-leg balancing squat with lateral rowing using a cable machine (use a band as an alternative); repeat on opposite leg
- Standing forward lunge with chest press; repeat on opposite leg
- Moving side squat with overhead press with low-weight dumbbell
- Medicine ball burpees (1 minute)
- Squat knee lift (alternating legs) (1 minute)
- Medicine ball burpees again for added intensity (1 minute)
- Tricep dips on bench (feet on floor or on top of stability ball)
- Standing lunge with lateral arm raise; repeat on opposite side
- Weighted squats
- Run or walk on treadmill or around track for 3-4 minutes
- Run in place holding medicine ball overhead (1 minute)
- Stand and rotate at the waist; hold cable or elastic band
- 5- to 10-minute cool down

Quick College Gym Workout

Equipment needed: a treadmill, exercise bike or elliptical machine

- 15 push-ups
- 20 burpees
- 10-minute walk or run on treadmill or track
- 10 push-ups
- 20 squat jumps
- 10 minutes on bike
- 15 tricep dips
- 15 lunges (each leg)
- 10 minutes on elliptical
- Repeat, if time allows

Basic Cardiovascular Workout

The following exercises are a great way to keep in shape, avoid gaining weight, and to feel healthy in college. Try to frequently change the exercise you do to keep things interesting and fun. All you need is 30-60 minutes.

- Run
- Walk
- Bike
- Elliptical
- Exercise class (cycling, step aerobics, kickboxing, etc.)
- Stairmaster (or climbing stairs)

Sometimes you may want to workout but feel too tired or have sore muscles. If that's the case, then mix it up by trying yoga, Pilates or just stretching in your dorm. Try the "College Yoga Flow" on page 180, designed for college women to build core strength and stretch their muscles. Remember, doing any form of fitness is always better than doing nothing.

One-Month Workout Plan

S	M	T	W	TH	F	S
	1 Cardio Bike Workout	**2** 60-Minute Gym Workout	**3** Go Running With Friend After Class	**4** 60-Minute Gym Workout	**5** Quick Dorm Room Workout	**6** Do "College Yoga Flow;" Bike For 20 – 30 minutes
7 DAY OFF	**8** Elliptical 30-60 Minutes	**9** Catch Cycling Class in After-noon	**10** Tough Gym Workout 60 Minutes	**11** Easy Cardio 30-Minute Workout	**12** Take Weight Lifting Class or do Dorm Workout	**13** Go Running With a Friend 30-60 Minutes
14 DAY OFF	**15** 60-Minute Gym Workout	**16** 30-Minute Easy Gym Workout	**17** 30-60 Minute Cardio Workout	**18** Workout in Dorm	**19** Bike to the Mall With a Friend	**20** DAY OFF
21 Walk Around Campus 30-60 Minutes	**22** Tough Gym Workout 60 Minutes	**23** Find a Yoga Class or Do Yoga in Dorm	**24** Elliptical 30-60 Minutes	**25** Tough Gym Workout 45 Minutes	**26** Run With a Friend After Class	**27** 30-Minute Core Workout in Dorm or Gym
28 DAY OFF	**29** Catch Cycling Class Before Class	**30** 45-Minute Easy Gym Workout	**31** Take Weight Lifting Class or Dorm Workout			

Chapter 6
Getting Enough Sleep

College is a lot of fun, with plenty of activities that will tempt you to stay up late into the night. Just trying to keep things in perspective can be tough, especially for freshmen. Too much fun and not enough sleep leads to fatigue, poor concentration, moodiness, stress, and illness. You need enough rest to do well in school, feel energized, and stay healthy, so make sure you try to find a balance in your time socializing, studying, and sleeping. That way, you can stay healthy and well rested, and enjoy all that college has to offer.

How Much Sleep Do I Need in College?
College-age women need seven or eight hours of sleep per night to be healthy, reduce stress, and feel energized in school.

Nine Healthy Sleep Habits

1. Try to sleep on a regular schedule. Whenever possible, get up and go to bed at the same time every day. The regularity of a sleep routine will help you fall asleep and feel more energetic in the morning.
2. Study ahead rather than cramming all night for an exam. Getting enough sleep the night before a test may improve your test-taking ability and help you maintain a regular sleep schedule. Steps for successful study habits are outlined in Chapter 23 to help you avoid "all-nighters."
3. Use your bed only for sleep. Do homework at your desk, not in your bed. Studying in bed may increase anxiety and brain activity when it's time to go to sleep, which can lead to insomnia.
4. Avoid working out during the three hours prior to bedtime because the adrenaline rush can keep you awake.
5. Minimize or avoid caffeinated beverages and food in the late afternoon and evening. Coffee, tea, chocolate, and pop contain caffeine, which increases your heart rate and brain stimulation and leads to difficulty falling sleep.
6. Do not eat a heavy meal just prior to bedtime because digestion or heartburn can keep you awake.

7. Talk to your roommate about boundaries and expectations. Agree on a schedule for quiet hours.
8. If you're feeling rundown, take a nap or get to bed earlier. Set your alarm so that the nap does not last longer than 30 minutes, and do not nap after 3 p.m. Sleeping too much midday interferes with nighttime sleep. Once you're feeling better, return to your regular sleep schedule.
9. Turn off all technology an hour before bedtime, if possible. Power down your phone so the sounds and lights do not bother or worry you and prevent you from sleeping. If you feel you need to keep your phone next to your bed, switch to "Airplane Mode" or turn on the "Do Not Disturb" setting.

What to Do If You Can't Sleep?
Try these Healthy Strategies for Insomnia

- If dorm noises prevent you from sleeping, invest in a small fan. The monotone sound of a running fan can drown out the background noise and create a peaceful environment for sleep. In addition, the fan will keep the room cool and comfortable, which can help you get to sleep.
- Load one of the helpful apps listed on the next page for relaxing melodies to create a calm and restful atmosphere for sleep.
- Try progressive muscle relaxation to help you get to sleep. Starting at your feet and moving upward through your body, relax each muscle group as you listen to the soothing sound of your fan or sleep app. Feel your legs, back, arms, neck, and head sink down into the mattress as you relax and fall asleep.
- Cut back on alcohol use. Alcohol can make you tired, but the quality of the sleep is often poor. Further, a hangover in the morning can make you feel sluggish throughout the day, which interferes with your schoolwork and nighttime sleep schedule.
- Try relaxing yoga poses just before bed to help you unwind and get some rest. There are steps for helpful poses in Chapter 21.
- Breathing techniques are beneficial for relaxation at bedtime. Steps are outlined in Chapter 22 to make it easy for you.
- Try acupuncture. There is literature in support of acupuncture to help with insomnia, but more research is needed. Be sure to find a qualified, board-certified acupuncturist.

<u>Helpful Apps</u> with good reviews:
Sleep Pillow Sounds, Relax Melodies, SleepBot, and Spotify

Nutritional Approach to Help You Sleep

- <u>Melatonin</u> is a natural hormone in your body that helps regulate sleep. Starting at dusk, melatonin levels naturally rise, and then taper down by the morning. There are many claims that supplemental melatonin can help with sleep, however, the literature on melatonin is mixed. Some studies say it works, and others say it does not. Melatonin supplements are available in tablet form over the counter, however, the FDA does not regulate the production, which can result in a slightly different amount of melatonin in each tablet. According to Mayo Clinic, the long-term safety of melatonin is not yet known, but it's generally thought to be safe to take for a few weeks. In order for melatonin to help you with sleep, the correct dosage needs to be taken at the correct time of day. Ask your doctor if this supplement is safe for you to try.
- <u>Chamomile tea</u>: Some people find a cup of chamomile tea relaxing and helpful for getting ready for sleep. Literature on chamomile tea is limited, and the production is not FDA-regulated. Roman chamomile is thought to help with sleep, however, its efficacy is not yet proven. As a caution, the pollen found in chamomile teas may cause allergic reactions and interfere with medications. If you are allergic to ragweed pollen, or taking blood thinner medications, do not try chamomile.

Caution About Using Over-the-Counter Sleep Aids

- <u>Antihistamines</u> are nonprescription allergy medications that some people take to make them feel drowsy and get to sleep.
- The problem with antihistamines is that they may initially make you groggy, but the quality of sleep is often poor, making you feel tired the next day.
- The side effects include confusion, daytime sleepiness, dizziness, nasal dryness, difficulty urinating, constipation, and dry mouth.
- It's better to try the "Healthy Strategies for Insomnia" to help you get to sleep rather than taking antihistamines.

- **Sleeping pills are dangerous medications and should not be taken unless prescribed by a doctor.** In my opinion, there are very few situations in which a sleeping pill is ever appropriate for a student. These medications make you less aware of what you are doing and more prone to dangerous situations. Further, sleeping pills can be addictive and make you psychologically dependent on the medication to sleep. **It is better to never start taking sleeping pills, and instead, figure out the reason for the insomnia and remove the cause.**

- It is very dangerous for women with **liver or kidney disease** to take sleeping pills because their bodies will not be able to break down the sleeping pill medications properly, making the sleeping pill's effect much stronger. These medications can further damage the liver and kidneys and increase the risk of an overdose and death.

- **Mixing sleeping pills with alcohol can be lethal. In other words, you can die if you mix sleeping pills and alcohol.** Even a small amount of alcohol can make you feel dizzy, weak, and confused after you have taken a sleeping pill. Do not drink any alcohol if you are taking sleeping pills.

- **If you want to stop taking sleeping pills, it is best to slowly wean off them as opposed to abruptly stopping.** There can be a sudden worsening of insomnia during the first week off the medication, if it is stopped too quickly. Be patient, and you will most likely return to a normal sleep pattern within a week of stopping the medication.

- **If your friend offers you a sleeping pill, say "NO."** Do not take anyone else's medications. If you can't sleep, and the strategies on page 60 do not work, call your doctor for help.

Chapter 7
What to Do If You Think You're Having a Medical Problem

Now that you're moving away from home, you are the one who's most responsible for your health. You need to be able to identify if you are having any of the common medical problems college women experience. You need to understand the basics about what is going on with your body and also recognize when you should seek medical advice.

The following chapters cover yeast infections, urinary tract/bladder infections, abnormal periods, iron-deficiency anemia, and depression. Each chapter will address the symptoms you may experience, risk factors, preventive measures, and common treatments. In addition, it will tell you when to go to the doctor or school health clinic.

It's important to understand that I'm not encouraging anyone to self-diagnose a condition. If you are worried about your health or have symptoms that are confusing or problematic, you should always seek medical advice from a professional.

Before College
1. Read the following chapters to become acquainted with several common medical conditions experienced by college women.

2. Program into your cell phone the following numbers:
   - Your family doctor
   - Your gynecologist
   - Your college's health services department

In College
1. Add the following numbers to your phone:
   - Your college counselor
   - The resident assistant in your dorm

2. If you are having **mild symptoms**, read through the following chapters to figure out what is possibly going on, what you can try to do on your own, and when to call the doctor or go to student health services.

3. If you are having more **severe symptoms**, or you've tried the suggestions in the following chapters and still have a problem, then you need to get help. The sooner you go, the faster you will feel better. Your family doctor, gynecologist, and school health service want to help you anytime you are having a problem - 24 hours a day, 7 days a week. Do not hesitate to call for help!

<u>Caution</u>

The information provided in this guidebook is to be used as a reference and is NOT intended to replace the medical advice of your doctor or healthcare provider. Please consult a professional for treatment if you are having a medical problem or need advice about any specific medical condition.

The sooner you seek help from your doctor for a medical problem, the better chance you have of fixing the problem and being healthy. Do not delay in calling the doctor or school health service if you are worried or confused about possibly having a medical problem.

Chapter 8
Yeast Infections

Yeast infections in the vagina, at the vaginal opening, and on the external genitalia are a very common condition. In fact, three out of four women will get a yeast infection in their lifetime.

What is it? Yeast is a fungus; it's a normal organism in the vagina in small amounts. A disruption of the normal vaginal pH allows the vaginal yeast to overgrow and cause symptoms.

Symptoms: An itching or burning sensation in the vagina or at the opening of the vagina, thick white discharge, and redness or swelling of the skin of the vulva (the external genitals) can all be symptoms of a yeast infection. Sometimes a patient will have all of these symptoms, while others experience only one.

Risk Factors for Yeast Infections
Recent antibiotics; diets high in sugar/sweets; alcohol; a suppressed immune system (possibly from getting worn down, pulling "all-nighters", and not getting enough sleep); higher-dose estrogen-containing birth control pills; inadequate lubrication (possibly from not drinking enough water); and douching (rinsing out the vagina, which strips the vagina of its normal pH balance).

When to See a Doctor
- If this is the first time you have experienced these symptoms
- If you are not sure if you have an infection
- If you've tried over-the-counter remedies, and they haven't been helpful

Treatment
- Over the counter: Monistat 3-Day Vaginal Cream or suppository can be purchased at any pharmacy without a prescription. I recommend the 3-Day treatment instead of the 1-Day treatment because it seems to be more effective for my patients. The cream and suppository both are equally effective, so pick whichever one you feel more comfortable using.

- Prescription Only:
    - o <u>Terazol</u> 3-Day Vaginal Cream or suppository
    - o <u>Diflucan</u> single oral tablet
    - o Your doctor, nurse practitioner or school health service will decide which of the above prescriptions is better for you. If you have a preference for oral versus vaginal treatment, be sure to mention it to the doctor or nurse.

Reduce Your Risk of Getting a Vaginal Yeast Infection

Avoid refined sugar; minimize alcohol; build your immune system with a healthy diet, exercise, and plenty of sleep; wear cotton underwear and loose fitting pants or skirts; avoid frequent use of thongs; change out of wet clothes, bathing suits, and Spandex shorts or pants as soon as possible; minimize use of hot tubs and very hot baths.

How to Avoid Getting Recurrent Yeast Infections

Avoid foods with a high mold or sugar content:

- Peanuts and pistachios
- Carbonated beverages
- Alcohol
- Milk
- Bananas
- Pineapples
- Fruit juices
- Potatoes
- White bread
- Aged cheeses
- Pickles
- Vinegars
- Mushrooms
- Sweets

Sometimes the Symptoms Are Not Due to Yeast

The following products can often give women an external irritation or internal "burning" that can be confused for a yeast infection:

- Liquid body washes
- Scented soaps (both liquid and bar form)
- Feminine sprays
- Cleansing wipes
- Lubricated condoms (contain Nonoxynol-9)
- Lubricants with a taste or that heat up

I find that my patients with symptoms of dryness, itching or irritation on the vulvar skin or vaginal opening seem to do the best with Dove-for-Sensitive-Skin Unscented Soap or Basis Soap, in bar form. These are just suggestions. See what works best for you.

Chapter 9
Bladder Infections
(Urinary Tract Infections)

Bladder infections are a very common condition in college. 25% of women beyond age 20 will have a bladder infection in their lifetime.

What is it?

A bladder infection is an overgrowth of bacteria inside the urinary tract, including the bladder, urethra, ureters and kidneys. Typically the urine inside is sterile, or free of bacteria. Occasionally, bacteria will ascend up the urethra into the bladder, causing an infection.

Typical Symptoms

- Pain with urination
- Strong urge to urinate
- Pressure sensation
- Cloudy urine
- Feeling that you have to urinate frequently but then not a lot of urine comes out

Some women experience only one symptom, while others suffer from many of the listed symptoms.

Symptoms of Severe Infection in the Bladder or Kidneys

- Bloody urine
- Fever
- Pain in the upper back

Risk Factors for Bladder Infections

- <u>Being female</u>: Bladder infections are more common in women than men as women have a shorter urethra, the tube that carries the urine from the bladder to the outside of the body.
- <u>Being sexually active</u>: Often the first bladder infection follows sexual activity. Some women feel like they have a bladder infection after each episode of intercourse.
- <u>Some types of birth control</u>: Nonoxynol-9, the spermicide in some lubricated condoms, diaphragms, and spermicidal jelly, can irritate the urethra and increase the risk of a bladder infection.
- <u>Suppressed immune system</u>: Being ill or getting rundown in school can make you more prone to infections.

When to See the Doctor

Contact the school health service or your doctor if you have any of the symptoms of a bladder infection listed on page 67.

Treatment

Antibiotics are a type of medicine that kill the bacteria that cause bladder infections. You will need a prescription from the school health service or your doctor for the antibiotic. Symptoms generally improve within two days, but be sure to complete the entire prescribed antibiotic or you risk the infection persisting and the symptoms returning quickly. If the bladder infection is severe or has traveled into the kidneys, you may need to stay in the hospital to be treated with more aggressive antibiotics.

Bladder Infections Following Intercourse

Some women complain that they routinely develop the symptoms of a bladder infection in the day or two following intercourse. Suggestions include:

- Have a urine culture to confirm if the symptoms are actually due to infection.
- Urinate before and after intercourse.
- Avoid the use of Nonoxynol-9 in spermicidal jelly and lubricated condoms. Use non-lubricated condoms instead.
- Consider taking a post-coital antibiotic, a single tablet of an antibiotic following intercourse to reduce the risk of a bladder infection specifically associated with intercourse. In order to find out if you qualify for this medical treatment, talk to your doctor.

How to Reduce the Risk of Developing a Bladder Infection

- Drink plenty of water to create more urine to flush out the bacteria.
- Minimize alcohol and caffeine; both can dehydrate your system.
- Urinate every three to four hours.
- Wipe from front to back to avoid transfer of bacteria from the anus to the urethra.
- Avoid the use of feminine powder and deodorant sprays.
- Drinking unsweetened cranberry juice or taking unsweetened cranberry pills may decrease the risk of symptomatic bladder infections, but according to Mayo Clinic, there is not enough

evidence to recommend its routine use to prevent bladder infections. Further, cranberry juice and tablets can upset the stomach, increase the risk of kidney stones, and be expensive.

Recurrent Bladder Infections

If you have more than three bladder infections in a year, you have met the criteria for what is called "Recurrent UTIs." For this circumstance, it is recommended that you see your doctor for further evaluation of what is causing the frequent problem.

Possible causes include:

- Anatomical abnormalities that you may have been born with
- Anatomical problems you may have developed over time
- Kidney stones

Once the evaluation has been done and the cause has been determined, your doctor can talk to you about the different options to help reduce your chance of a recurrent bladder infection.

Options to Ease the Discomfort of a Bladder Infection

- Avoid food and drinks that irritate the bladder (see the "Common Bladder Irritants List" on the next page).
- Try a heating pad.
- Avoid potentially irritating feminine products such as feminine sprays, powders, and wipes that can irritate the urethra.
- Drink water to dilute the urine and flush out bacteria.
- Talk to your doctor about prescription medications for bladder discomfort or pain.

Food and Drinks that Bother the Bladder:
A Bladder Irritants List

This is a list of common foods and beverages that can irritate the bladder and worsen the symptoms during a bladder infection. Further, these irritants can cause symptoms that mimic an infection. If you have a bladder infection, avoid the food and drinks on this list until you've completed medical treatment and the bladder symptoms have gone away. If you "always have a bladder infection," it may be a food or drink in your diet that irritates the bladder and mimics the symptoms of an infection. Try to identify the irritant to avoid it and feel better.

Common Bladder Irritants List

Alcohol
Caffeine: coffee, tea, pop, and chocolate
Carbonated beverages: pop, diet pop, tonic, and seltzer
Sugar and sugar substitutes
Tomatoes
Vinegar
Spicy food
Citrus juices
Peaches
Plums
Strawberries
Cantaloupe
Apples
Grapes
Guava
Pineapple
B-complex vitamins

You don't have to stop consuming everything on this list at one time. Instead, keep a diary of everything you eat and drink from this list over a two-week period of time. Write down which days your symptoms are worse than others so you can identify a pattern, such as cantaloupe or caffeinated beverages. Once you understand what dietary product is bothersome to your bladder, minimize or eliminate that particular irritant from your diet to avoid the symptoms.

If you love something from this list but it annoys your bladder, avoid it when you have something important to do. On days you will be hanging out in your dorm and able to go to the bathroom more frequently, feel free to enjoy it. Understanding what irritates your bladder will help you feel comfortable and more in control.

Chapter 10
Abnormal Periods

Abnormal periods are a common problem for college women. Approximately 15-20% of college-age women will develop an abnormal menstrual cycle at some time during their four years in school.

Is My Period Normal?

The menstrual cycle starts on the first day of menstrual flow. A normal menstrual cycle ranges from 21-35 days (from the first day of one period to first day of next), and lasts up to seven days.

- Most women have periods about every 28 days, lasting between four and seven days.
- Most say the flow is light on the first day, heavier on the second day, and then tapers down from there.
- Many women have brown or red spotting the day before the flow starts or a few days after the flow ends.
- Any version of a flow is fine as long as it does not meet the definition of abnormal bleeding described below.

What is an Abnormal Period?

Any of the following situations is abnormal:

- A period that starts sooner than 21 days since the *first day* of the last menstrual period
- When the period starts further than 35 days since the *first day* of the last period
- If the flow of the period lasts longer than seven days
- If the flow is heavy with clots
- Anytime there is bleeding between the periods
- Anytime there is significant pain associated with the period
- Anytime there is bleeding after intercourse

How Do I Know if My Period is Abnormally Heavy?

- If you need double protection: tampon and pad, or two pads
- If you change your tampon or pad in the middle of the night
- If you soak through a tampon or pad every hour for several hours in a row

Terms to Describe Abnormal Periods

- Amenorrhea: when the period stops for three or more months
- Oligomenorrhea: when periods are farther apart than 35 days
- Menorrhagia: when the period is very heavy or lasts longer than seven days
- Metrorrhagia: when the period is irregular in timing and "comes whenever it wants"
- Dysmenorrhea: painful periods or severe menstrual cramps

Keep Track of Your Period

- Always write down the *first day of your menstrual period*. It is used to calculate if your periods are normal or not. Further, if you get pregnant, the doctor will need this information to figure out how far along the pregnancy is.
- Also keep track of the number of days between your periods, how heavy the flow is, and how long the flow lasts. The doctor will want this information.

Helpful Apps

My patients often prefer to use an app to record their periods, and many suggest the following two apps:

- Clue period tracker
- Period Tracker ("P-Tracker")

When to See the Doctor

It is perfectly normal for most women to experience an abnormal cycle occasionally. Just be sure to confirm that you are not pregnant. Be patient, and your periods will most likely return to normal within two cycles. If your periods continue to be abnormal for more than two cycles in a row, you need to see a doctor.

If you might be pregnant, have heavy periods, experience severe menstrual pain or bleeding after intercourse, then see a doctor right away.

A doctor will do a physical exam, some blood tests, genital cultures, and may order an ultrasound to diagnose the reason for your abnormal periods. The following pages outline several causes of abnormal periods.

Common Causes of Abnormal Periods

- Pregnancy: One of the leading causes of an abnormal period is pregnancy. If you have been sexually active and have an irregular period, you must take a pregnancy test. You can buy an inexpensive test at the pharmacy.
- Excessive weight loss or gain: Being underweight (BMI<18.5) is a common cause of missed or irregular periods; obesity (BMI>29) can also cause irregular periods. Refer to the BMI chart in Chapter 3 for a healthy target weight range.
- Eating disorders: Anorexia and bulimia can cause a change in the menstrual cycle. See Chapter 3 for information.
- Increased exercise: Irregular periods are common in athletes.
- Emotional stress: Research is limited on the impact of stress on menstruation, but there is an association of abnormal periods and women with premenstrual syndrome (PMS) or depression.
- Birth control pills (OCPs): OCPs may cause the period to lighten, spot or skip all together. Refer to info about OCPs in Chapter 14.
- Hormone problems: Women with thyroid disease can also have irregular periods.

Specific Gynecologic Conditions that Cause Abnormal Periods

- Polycystic Ovarian Syndrome
  A condition in which the ovaries do not ovulate consistently, causing a woman to skip periods or not have periods at all. The ovaries of patients with PCOS make an excessive amount of male hormones causing acne, oily skin, and facial hair. Some patients may develop a metabolic problem, called insulin resistance, and have problems with their weight and be at an increased risk of diabetes. The exact reason for PCOS is not known, but patients with PCOS and insulin resistance can benefit from OCPs, weight loss, exercise, and a diet aimed at avoiding refined sugar. Occasionally, patients need additional medications including spironolactone and metformin.

- Endometriosis
  A condition when the menstrual blood and tissue get into the pelvis rather than flushing out with the period. The exact cause is not known, but a common theory is that the blood and tissue back up from the uterus, through the fallopian tubes and into the pelvis. The tissue then implants on the other organs in the pelvis,

grows, bleeds, and eventually scars. Endometriosis can lead to painful, heavy periods and painful intercourse for many patients. In addition, it can cause infertility. If you have painful, heavy periods, get an evaluation for endometriosis by your doctor. The first line of treatment is usually birth control pills (OCPs) and Ibuprofen. If these treatments are not helpful, laparoscopic surgery or medications to temporarily stop your hormones is the next step to diagnosing and treating endometriosis.

- Fibroids
  A fibroid is an overgrowth of the muscle in the uterus, typically shaped into a ball. These common tumors are rarely cancerous, but can cause heavy or irregular periods. The fibroids themselves do not typically cause pain, but can push on the bladder or rectum and cause a sense of pressure. You do not need treatment for the fibroids unless they grow very large or protrude into the cavity of the uterus, causing abnormal periods.

- Uterine polyps
  Uterine polyps are an overgrowth of the lining of the uterus, typically shaped into an oval. These common tumors are rarely cancerous, but can cause bleeding between the periods or after intercourse. Your doctor will recommend whether to observe the polyps, start medical treatment or surgically remove them.

- Ovarian cysts
  An ovarian cyst is a "fluid-filled ball" that grows in an ovary. You have normal cysts in your ovaries called follicles that contain your eggs and enable you to get pregnant someday. Abnormal ovarian cysts form when your hormones are imbalanced. Less commonly, some cysts grow and need to be removed surgically. Ovarian cancer can happen in young women, but it is not common. Women with ovarian cysts can complain of pelvic pain, pelvic pressure or irregular periods. The most common treatment for cysts is to start OCPs. If the cyst is large, has a "complex" look on ultrasound, persists for several months or causes significant pain, the patient may need to have it surgically removed. Once an ovarian cyst is diagnosed, your doctor can recommend the best type of treatment.

- Anovulation
  A condition when the ovaries are not working properly. Women with this problem do not ovulate each month and, therefore, do not have their period every month. This is usually due to an immature neurologic pathway in young women, and will most likely normalize with time and not require treatment. OCPs can be used to start to regulate the menstrual cycle.

- Pelvic Inflammatory Disease
  A severe form of a sexually transmitted infection that has spread up into the uterus, fallopian tubes, and into the pelvis. It can cause the patient to have abundant discharge, odor, pain, fever, nausea, and an abnormal period. PID can be life-threatening if it's not treated. It can also cause scarring in the fallopian tubes, which can cause long-term pain and can prevent pregnancy in the future (infertility). The treatment for PID is antibiotics, frequently given at a hospital. Condoms can minimize the risk of PID by preventing contact with sexually transmitted infections.

A good resource for questions or concerns and a more in-depth explanation regarding these gynecologic conditions can be found on the American Congress of OB/GYNE website: http://www.acog.org/Patients

---

Final Thoughts

- Most likely, an abnormal period is not due to anything serious and will correct itself over time.
- If you have *ever* been sexually active in *any way*, you need to take a pregnancy test.
- If you are not sexually active, be patient, and your periods will most likely return to normal within two cycles.
- If the abnormal periods persist more than two cycles, you should see a doctor for an evaluation.
- If you have pain with your periods or bleeding after intercourse, call your doctor right away.
- Remember the above guidelines are just a rule of thumb. Always seek medical advice from your doctor or school health service any time you have concern that your period is not normal.

Service to Others

Think about the millions of girls and women around the world who do not have access to menstrual pads, clean toilets or running water. In many countries, it is shameful to get your period, so girls hide it. Without access to menstrual hygiene necessities, many girls don't go to school during the week of their period and therefore miss out on their education. Menstrual pads and toilets are taken for granted by many of us but are an unmet necessity by millions of others. Consider getting involved and supporting one of these organizations:

1. **AFRIpads Ltd.**
Located in Uganda, this business "manufactures and sells cost-effective cloth sanitary pads. AFRIpads are washable, cloth sanitary pads designed to provide effective and hygienic menstrual protection for up to one year (12 cycles) at a fraction of the cost of an equivalent supply of disposable pads. The innovative product design is comfortable, cost-saving, and environmentally-friendly." www.afripads.com

2. **UNICEF**
This organization supports humanitarian issues worldwide and has taken action to address the menstrual hygiene management challenges that are faced by schoolgirls throughout the world. UNICEF "fosters social inclusion and individual self-respect," and provides education and support in Afghanistan, Pakistan, India, Africa, the Philippines and many other countries. www.unicef.org

3. **Women in Europe for a Common Future**
This organization is an "international network of over 150 women's, environmental, and health organizations working on projects in 50 countries." WECF's school toilet program provides access for menstrual hygiene and safe and sustainable sanitation for women throughout Europe.
http://www.wecf.eu/english/campaigns/2012/Sustainable_Sanitation_for_Women.php

Chapter 11
Iron Deficiency Anemia

Iron deficiency anemia is a common medical condition in college-age women. In the United States, 6 million reproductive-age women are iron deficient, and approximately 50 percent of these women will become anemic.

What is it?

Iron deficiency anemia is defined as a low blood count caused by not having enough iron in your body. Iron is needed to make healthy red blood cells, which carry oxygen throughout your body.

Common Symptoms

- Fatigue, or feeling tired all the time, is the most common symptom.
- Headaches are a complaint many of my patients have when they are anemic.
- Looking pale. Don't panic if you are pale naturally.
- Dizziness, weakness or shortness of breath
- Brittle nails
- Cold hands and feet
- Heart palpitations

Less Common Complaints

- Pica: craving ice
- Restless Leg Syndrome: a tingling or "crawling" feeling in your legs
- Feeling depressed

Causes

- Heavy or Long Menstrual Periods: 10-15 percent of women have heavy periods. Of these women, 20 percent will become anemic.
    - o Periods that last longer than seven days
    - o Needing to use double protection (tampon plus pad or two pads)
    - o Passing large blood clots with your period
    - o Having to change your tampon or pad during the night

- Soaking through your tampon and/or pad every hour for several hours in a row
- Inadequate iron intake: A poor diet among college students is a common cause of iron deficiency anemia.
- Low calorie intake: Inadequate calorie intake causing a low body weight can lead to anemia. Being "underweight" is defined as a Body Mass Index less than 18.5. People on diets and those with eating disorders frequently have anemia.
- Less common causes: Celiac disease, kidney problems, and some forms of cancer can lead to anemia.

Who is at Risk?
- Women are at risk due to menstruation.
- College students are at risk due to poor nutrition and inadequate iron intake.
- Athletes are especially at risk due to inadequate iron intake, poor iron absorption, increased red blood cell destruction, and loss of iron in perspiration and in the intestinal tract. The symptoms of anemia are more common for athletes due to low iron storage levels and the increased oxygen demand required for exercise.

When to See the Doctor
If you feel tired and rundown, look pale, or feel weak or dizzy, call your doctor for a check-up. Iron deficiency anemia is one possible cause of these symptoms, and your doctor will evaluate you.

Blood Tests Your Doctor Will Order
- Complete Blood Count: checks the level of hemoglobin in your blood which carries the oxygen throughout your body
- Iron Level: measures the amount of iron in your body
- Ferritin level: indicates the amount of iron stored in your body for future use
- Other blood tests to make sure your symptoms are not caused by a different medical condition

How to Prevent Iron Deficiency Anemia
- Talk to your doctor if you have heavy periods; reducing the amount of menstrual flow each month can help you avoid and treat anemia. OCPs are the usual treatment to make your periods

shorter and lighter. Typically, your period will only last two or three days and be very light. The other treatment option to lighten the menstrual flow is a hormonal intrauterine device. Talk to your doctor about which option is best for you. See Chapter 14 for additional information.

- Be sure to get enough iron. The recommended daily iron you need is 15-18 mg. Eat plenty of iron-rich foods listed below, or buy an iron supplement. If you have food sensitivities, look for a vitamin that is free of artificial flavors, colors, and preservatives; the local whole food market will sell an iron supplement free of these additives. Talk to your doctor before taking any supplement.
- Get enough vitamin C to help your body absorb the iron. It's best to consume vitamin C at the same time that you consume iron for the best absorption. You need 65-75 mg vitamin C daily.
- If you are anemic, avoid food that block the absorption of iron, including tannic acid in tea and polyphenol in coffee.

Foods that Contain Iron

- Red meat
- Pork
- Chicken
- Seafood
- Liver
- Dried fruit, such as raisins and apricots
- Cereals fortified with iron
- Bread fortified with iron
- Dark green, leafy veggies, such as spinach
- Peas
- Beans

The iron in meat, chicken, pork and seafood is absorbed better than iron from fruit, veggies, fortified cereals and breads.

Foods that Contain Vitamin C

- Oranges/Tangerines
- Strawberries
- Grapefruit/Melons
- Kiwi
- Broccoli
- Green leafy veggies
- Tomatoes
- Peppers

Iron can cause constipation
What you can do:

Constipation is defined as having less than 3 bowel movements per week. Constipation can make you feel uncomfortable or cause you to strain to have a bowel movement.

- Increase your fiber intake through fruits and veggies. According to Mayo Clinic, you need approximately 14 grams of fiber for every 1000 calories. Start slowly because too much fiber too quickly can cause bloating.
- Drink plenty of water to keep the stool soft.
- Exercise daily to help the muscles of the intestines function better.
- Try foods that soften the stool such as prunes and dried apricots.
- If you are taking an iron supplement and feeling constipated, try a stool softener from the local pharmacy twice per week. Look on the bottle to be sure you are purchasing a stool softener, not a stimulating laxative.
- If you are struggling with constipation and none of the ideas above are helpful, see the doctor. Do not take stimulating laxatives unless recommended by your doctor.

Final Thoughts

Iron deficiency anemia is common in college. If you are experiencing dizziness, headaches, fatigue, heavy periods or any of the symptoms listed above, be sure to talk to your doctor or the student health service to be evaluated for iron deficiency anemia.

Chapter 12
Depression

According to the National Institute on Mental Health, "depression is a common but serious mental illness typically marked by sad or anxious feelings. Most college students occasionally feel sad or anxious, but these emotions usually pass quickly—within a couple of days. Untreated depression lasts for a long time, interferes with day-to-day activities, and is much more than just being 'a little down' or 'feeling blue.'" All of the following depression information comes directly from the NIMH website:

How does Depression Affect College Students?

- 30% of college students reported feeling "so depressed that it was difficult to function" at some time in the past year.
- Depression can affect academic performance in college.
- College students who have depression are more likely to smoke.
- Students with depression do not necessarily drink alcohol more heavily than other college students, but students with depression, especially women, are more likely to drink to get drunk and experience problems related to alcohol abuse, such as engaging in unsafe sex.
- Depression often co-occurs with substance abuse, which can complicate treatment.

Depression is also a Major Risk Factor for Suicide

- More than 6% of college students have reported seriously considering suicide.
- 1% of college students have reported attempting suicide in the previous year.
- Suicide is the third-leading cause of death for teens and young adults ages 15-24.
- Warning signs for depression in men can be different than the warning signs for women.
- Better diagnosis and treatment of depression can help reduce suicide rates among college students.

What Causes Depression?

- Depression does not have a single cause. Several factors can lead to depression.
- Some people carry genes that increase their risk of depression. But not all people with depression have these genes, and not all people with these genes have depression.
- Environment—surroundings and life experiences, such as stress, can contribute to depression.

Six College-related Stresses that can Lead to Depression

1. Living away from family for the first time
2. Missing family or friends
3. Feeling alone or isolated
4. Experiencing conflict in relationships
5. Facing new and sometimes difficult school work
6. Worrying about finances

What are the Signs and Symptoms of Depression?

The symptoms vary, so if you are depressed, you may feel:

- Sad, anxious, empty, hopeless, guilty, worthless, helpless, irritable, and restless
- Loss of interest in activities you used to enjoy
- Lack of energy
- Problems concentrating, remembering information or making decisions
- Problems falling asleep, staying asleep or sleeping too much
- Loss of appetite or eating too much
- Thoughts of suicide or suicide attempts
- Aches, pains, headaches, cramps or digestive problems that do not go away

How do I Know if I have Depression, and Where can I get Help?

- The first step is to talk with a doctor or mental health care provider. Your family doctor, campus health center staff or other trusted adult may be able to help you find appropriate care.
- Most colleges provide mental health services through counseling centers, student health centers, or both. Student health centers provide basic health care services to students at little or no cost. Check out your college website for information.

How is Depression Treated?

- Common treatments are antidepressants and psychotherapy.
- A doctor or mental health care provider can help find the treatment that's right for you.

How can I Help Myself if I am Depressed?

- The first step to feeling better is to call your doctor or school health service to get help. Try to see a professional as soon as possible—research shows that getting treatment sooner rather than later can relieve symptoms quicker and reduce the length of time treatment is needed.
- Give treatment a fair chance—attend sessions and follow your doctor or therapist's advice, including advice about specific exercises or "homework" to try between appointments.
- Break up large tasks into small ones, and do what you can as you can; try not to do too many things at once.
- Spend time with other people and talk to a friend or relative about your feelings.
- Do not make important decisions until you feel better; talk about decisions with others whom you trust and who know you well
- Engage in mild exercise, and participate in activities that you used to enjoy.
- Expect your mood to improve gradually with treatment.
- Remember that positive thinking will replace negative thoughts as your depression responds to treatment.
- For more information, visit the website: www.nimh.nih.gov.

What if I am in Crisis? What if Someone I Know is in Crisis?

- Call your doctor or mental health care provider.
- Call 911 or go to a hospital emergency room to get immediate help, or ask a friend or family member to help you do these things.
- Call your campus suicide or crisis hotline, counseling center or student health service.
- Call the National Suicide Prevention Lifeline 1-800-273-TALK (1-800-273-8255) or TTY 1-800-799-4TTY (1-800-799-4889) to talk to a trained counselor.
- If you are in crisis, make sure you are not left alone.
- If someone else is in crisis, make sure he or she is not left alone.

As indicated above, the information in this chapter came directly from the National Institute of Mental Health. For more information about depression, visit www.nimh.nih.gov.

Other Helpful Resources

- *The Jed & Clinton Health Matters Campus Program (The Campus Program)* is a program "designed to help colleges and universities assess and enhance mental health, substance abuse, and suicide prevention programming."
  http://www.jedfoundation.org

- *ULifeline* has helpful information and an online mental health evaluator
  http://www.ulifeline.org

Be Safe

One young woman, in her sophomore year of college, was walking home through the parking lot of her college gym after working out and was attacked by a guy who was hiding between two cars. It was dark outside, the parking lot had dim lighting, and she was alone. She didn't see the attacker crouched down until she was right next to the cars where he was hiding. He grabbed her arm and said in a low voice, "You're not leaving until I ---- you" and began to pull her down between the cars. She could hear other people across the parking lot, so she tried to yell for help, but sound wouldn't come out of her mouth. The only thing she could think of doing was to try to kick at him before he could get her all the way down onto the ground. After a few quick tries, one of her kicks landed hard on his knee. He released his grip enough that she was able to twist and run away. She quickly caught up to the people who had been walking nearby, not joining their group, but quietly walking behind as if she was just another student walking home. Feeling shocked and afraid, she didn't tell them what had happened. In fact, she didn't tell anyone about the assault initially, not even her family. After that night, she was very frightened to walk through campus, and no longer worked out at the gym.

Many of my patients have told me that they have had similar incidences to this during their years in college. I can relate to how frightening their experiences must have been because I was the woman in this story. I'm thankful that I was able to get away without being raped, but not every woman is so lucky.

I learned a lot that night about the world and how other people could affect me. Although my college campus was a beautiful place with plenty of nice people, and a great place for learning, it couldn't guarantee my safety. No college could.

I knew it wasn't my fault that I was attacked, and that the guy was morally and legally wrong, but the experience made me think a lot about how I wanted to move forward in my life. I realized that I needed to take steps to be safer on campus and to protect myself. Although no one ever really feels prepared to be attacked, there were things I could have done differently that would have made my college experience safer for me. I should not have been walking home alone at night, especially in a dimly lit parking lot. I should have had a whistle on my key chain or been able to scream out if I needed help. My biggest realization was that I should have taken a self-defense class before I was attacked.

Looking back on my recovery from that night, I realize that it would have been healthier for me to have told someone about what had happened to me. I had a strong sense of self, even at a young age, and I was able to move forward, but not without a lot of fear for many years. Counseling at that time would have been helpful for my healing. Further, had I told the police, perhaps the guy would have been caught so he couldn't hurt anyone else.

There were several changes I made in my life after that experience. I began to plan ahead to coordinate my schedule with my friends and walk through campus in a group of people, especially at night. I put a whistle on my key chain, and memorized the campus bus schedule. Although I would only workout in my dorm room from that point on, at least I was taking steps to heal. In addition, I joined a taekwondo class to learn self-defense and to practice yelling out loud. These steps may not have been completely effective in some situations, but they made me feel more powerful and more aware of my capabilities to protect myself.

Years later, I am a gynecologist taking care of young women about to head off to college, and I want them to be safe. I want to give them my perspective to help them be prepared for what is ahead. Most of my patients have great experiences in college, but I've treated many young women with problems along the way, and realize that college-bound women need to learn how to be safe before they leave home.

Safety is not just learning ways to avoid sexual assault or taking a self-defense class. It is also about making good choices with regards to your sexuality, preventing unplanned pregnancy, and avoiding sexually transmitted diseases.

In addition, safety means not taking drugs even when other people tell you that the drugs are OK because a doctor prescribes them.

I have written the following chapters to give you the information you need to understand the social and health issues you will encounter away from home. Think about your personal values as you apply this information to your life. The following chapters are possibly intimidating to you, but I don't want you to be afraid. Instead, I want you to have a clear understanding about what you will be facing in college, and the tools to handle these situations in the safest way. Being prepared can help you be safe, stay on track with school, and take good care of yourself when you move out on your own.

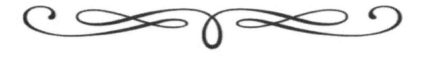

"I find the women who have a solid sense of self, including their personal values, seem to make healthier lifestyle choices in college."

-M. Susan Scanlon, M.D.
The Gyne's Guide

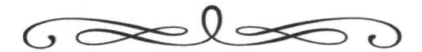

Chapter 13
Let's Talk About Sex

Every year, I extend my office hours on the Friday and Saturday after Thanksgiving to take care of the college women coming home who've had problems. It's typically freshmen who need the appointments, and the reasons for the visits are often related to sexuality.

Sex

The topic of sexuality seems to be an intriguing subject for many people. Books are written, movies created, and songs sung. Sexual expression seems to be all around us. Although some people may want to tell you what you should think and do with regards to your sexuality, in the end the decision is completely up to you.

I encourage you to give serious thought to your personal values and how you feel about sexuality *before* you go to college. No pressure. No judgment. No quick decisions or random choices. Just some serious consideration about who you really are and what you feel is important to you. This thoughtful approach is an important part of getting prepared for college and deciding how you will handle things when you're away from home. As a gynecologist, I find that the women who have a solid sense of self, including their personal values, seem to make healthier lifestyle choices in college. They also seem happier with the outcomes of their decisions.

College is going to present you with abundant freedom to do whatever you want and with whomever you want. Perhaps you feel experienced with dating, but most likely in high school you had to be accountable to your parents or another adult. In college, you will need to be accountable to yourself. Without a solid sense of who you really are, you may find yourself in a circumstance of randomly taking an action that is not consistent with the woman you want to be, and then ultimately feeling bad about your choice. Equally as problematic, poor planning can lead to an unwanted pregnancy or a sexually transmitted disease.

Planning ahead on how you want to handle the different social situations you will face in college will prepare YOU to be healthy, safe and happy when away from home.

Emma

Emma came home from college for the Thanksgiving holiday and made an appointment to come into my office. She was worried that she could be pregnant or have an STD. She had gone with her girl-friends to a party the weekend before and had sex with a guy who she did not really know.

Emma told me that she had started to drink beer in high school, but as a freshman in college, she began drinking hard alcohol and frequently got drunk. At the party, she met a guy she liked who was friendly and nice, so she decided to "do shots" of raspberry vodka with him. After a while, Emma knew she was getting drunk, but she was having fun, and she didn't really care.

Eventually, Emma was intoxicated, and she lost her sense of control. The next morning, she woke up in the guy's dorm room and had to walk home in the clothes she wore out the night before. She felt humiliated in front of her roommate because she didn't come home the night before and didn't know the name of guy she had stayed with. Even worse, she thought she had intercourse, but wasn't sure, and she had no idea if they used a condom. She was worried that she was exposed to an STD or could be pregnant. Emma said she felt bad about her decisions to drink so much and to stay with a strange guy.

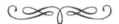

Lindsey

Lindsey came into the office on the weekend following Thanksgiving. She was tearful and expressed that she was upset about something that had happened in college. One girl from her dorm challenged all the girls to a contest to see how many guys they could "sleep with" over one month. Lindsey wanted to make friends and "fit in," and decided that she would agree to participate, but would pretend that she was doing it. She didn't realize that the guy she would invite over wasn't pretending, and he would pressure her to have sex. She just thought he would hang out. He had other ideas. He didn't bring a condom, and one thing led to another, and she agreed to have unprotected sex. Lindsey felt completely overwhelmed in college. She realized she was making random decisions, and she really didn't know why.

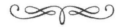

A *Gynecologist's Perspective*

Every year, there are countless patient stories similar to these that I could tell. Both Emma and Lindsey are nice women with wonderful goals for themselves. Both want to have healthy relationships and feel good about their college experience. Unfortunately, both made decisions without enough thought in advance and were unhappy with the outcomes of their actions. This problem is common for my college-age patients and is one of the most important reasons I've written this guidebook.

As a gynecologist, I have a unique perspective of the challenges you may face in college, and I want you to have the information you need to be on top of it all. I recommend that you think through your views on sexuality BEFORE moving away from home and then revisit the topic as you navigate your way over the following four years. Most importantly, make choices consistent with the woman you want to be. You will not always be perfect, but if you can follow this approach, you will stay on track to be your best and to be happy with the outcomes of your decisions.

Basic Facts about Sexuality

- Approximately 80% of women will have sex during college.
- 80% of sexually active college women do not consistently use contraception and therefore put themselves at risk of unplanned pregnancy.
- The unwanted pregnancy rate in the United States is 50%.
- Of 18- and 19-year-old women, 83% of pregnancies are unintended.

- Of 20- to 24-year-old women, 64% of pregnancies are unintended.
- 10% of college women will become pregnant.
- The risk of unwanted pregnancy increases with binge drinking.

Questions to Consider About Your Sexuality

Whenever one of my patients comes into the office because she has decided to become sexually active, I ask her a few questions to help her solidify her thoughts about her sexuality. I'd encourage you to ask yourself these same questions:

- Are you starting to have sex because it's something you want to do, something you feel you're supposed to do or something you're doing because you fear the guys won't like you if you don't?
- Do you feel that you're emotionally ready for a sexual relationship? Is the person you are choosing to have sex with kind and respectful of you?
- If you're deciding to become sexually active, are you going to be monogamous or will you be experimenting with multiple partners?
- Have you thought through how you're going to protect yourself against pregnancy and sexually transmitted diseases?

One area that is often difficult for young women to come to terms with is when their religious beliefs come into conflict with their sexual choices. If this is the case in your life, you will need to think about how you will cope with this conflict. If you make choices outside of your religious foundation, how will that make you feel? The ideal time to address this conflict is *before you start to have sex*. If you've already become sexually active and have never given it thought, review in your mind how you feel and then decide if you will continue or make any changes. This is a very private and personal decision that only you can make and it is not for me or anyone else to judge. I would just encourage you to think it through.

Taking Responsibility

As a gynecologist, I tell my patients that sex is an adult activity. Therefore, if you're going to have sex, be a responsible adult by being prepared. Use contraception to prevent an unplanned pregnancy and protect yourself against sexually transmitted diseases. Furthermore, wait to have sex until you are emotionally ready to take on a sexual relationship.

If you've done something sexually that you have later regretted, then learn from it, forgive yourself, and move forward in a new direction. Remember that everyone has made mistakes, and you're not the only one who is trying to figure things out. Next time, think about what you are choosing to do BEFORE taking action. This will give you the best chance of being happy with the outcomes of your choices.

Self-Esteem and Sexuality

The concept of self-esteem has been researched since the 1960s, and studies published by Silber and Tippett described self-esteem as "the feelings a person has about (herself) that reflect the relationship between the self-image and the ideal self-image." In other words, your self-esteem depends on how you actually see yourself compared to how you would ideally like to see yourself. A woman with low self-esteem does not see herself measuring up to what she wants to be. A different woman who has high self-esteem sees herself as meeting her best vision of herself.

How does this affect your sexuality? Some research has shown that women with lower self-esteem and lower self-awareness oftentimes have higher rates of sexual activity. Maybe these women are looking for approval. Maybe they're lonely. Maybe they just want to be loved and don't realize that sex is not the way to get love. There are many theories, but the important thing is to recognize that your self-esteem can be impacted by the choices you make about sexuality. I have observed that my patients who randomly or carelessly have sex often do not feel good about themselves afterwards. Many say that they wished that they had waited to have sex until there was some important significance in their relationship. Before you have sex, be absolutely sure that you want to be intimate with the person you are about to have sex with, and that the emotional component of having sex is worth it to you. Keep in mind the impact your choices can have on your self-esteem. Having a strong sense of self is not often easy but definitely worth working on.

Dating Does Not Equal Sex

Starting a new relationship is exciting for all women. Going out on dates helps you to figure out what kind of person you are compatible with, as well as to find someone who shares your same values. Look around carefully and see what there is to offer! Understand, though, that dating and sex are not the same thing. You can date, get to know each other, and have fun without having sex. Don't let anyone fool you---just because you are dating doesn't mean you have to have sex.

You get to choose when sex is appropriate based on your personal values and the relationship you are in. Think carefully about how a sexual relationship will impact you both physically and emotionally *before you have sex.*

As a gynecologist, I have taken care of women who have decided to have sex just to "get a guy to like them" or because they "thought it was expected." Other patients have had sex with several different partners "because everyone does." Many times these women had a hard time coping with the emotional let-down when the sexual relationship did not evolve into something more meaningful.

The bottom line is this...if your new boyfriend pressures you to have sex when you're not ready, be strong and say "No!" Recognize that YOU are valuable and your sexuality is important. If he can't respect how you feel, I encourage you to respect yourself by finding a different boyfriend.

Choosing a Partner

If you do decide to become sexually active, make sure that the partner you're picking is worth sharing your sexuality with. Is he kind and respectful of you? Do you feel positive and comfortable with him? Think carefully about the values this new partner has....are they similar to yours?

On the other hand, if the new partner disrespects you, uses you, pressures you, hurts you, gets you drunk, embarrasses you, shames you or takes advantage of you—I'd encourage you to break up with him and move on. There are millions of guys to choose from. Why settle for someone who is not worthy of what you have to offer?

Oral Sex

An issue I see as a gynecologist is that many college-age women seem to think that having oral sex is not sex. Because they don't view it as sex, some women will have oral sex casually, often with no intention of a relationship or even knowing their partner. As a gynecologist, I can assure you that this view about oral sex is not accurate. Any form of sexual activity is having sex, including both giving and receiving oral sex, and puts you at risk for the emotional and physical consequences of sexual activity.

Many patients who have had oral sex with random people tell me they feel bad about what they did. "I knew I shouldn't have been doing that." Many say that they feel like they've been used and don't feel good about it. Other patients face the upsetting fact that they've been exposed to an STD in their mouth, like herpes or chlamydia.

Before you choose to have oral sex with someone, think it through carefully. Is it something you want to do? Are you doing it just because you think you're supposed to? Do you feel pressure from friends to give or receive oral sex? I encourage you to reserve sex, including oral sex, for a special monogamous relationship rather than a casual or random encounter. Don't let someone pressure you into it. Be sure you're emotionally ready for the choice you're making and protect yourself from oral STDs. I have found that the patients who have taken this approach seem to be happiest with their decisions.

Feeling Empowered

Some patients tell me that they like to have sex because it makes them feel powerful. My question to them is, "Do you think sex is about a mutual respectful relationship with someone or do you thinks it's about having power over someone else?"

I would challenge you to actually be empowered by holding off from having sex, avoiding multiple partners, and considering abstinence until you know with certainty that you have found a truly meaningful relationship based on common values. That's the actual power you could demonstrate. True empowerment comes from choosing a healthy approach to your sexuality, both emotionally and physically, and making decisions consistent with the woman you want to be.

What to Do if You Change Your Mind?

Sometimes, even with the best of intentions and planning, circumstances can change in a way that you didn't expect. It's important to be able to get out of a situation that is going in a direction that makes you feel uncomfortable or is unsafe for you to be in. Be prepared in advance of the situation so that you can handle it with confidence.

The first thing to do is to say, "NO!" and get up to leave. No matter what is said to try to sway your decision, stay strong and firm and move away from the situation. In addition, I would suggest that you have a few sentences in mind that you can say that can put a stop to a bad situation before things get worse. Then practice your sentences in advance so they're easy for you draw upon when it's time.

Suggested Sentences to Stop a Bad Situation from Getting Worse

Based on my experience as a gynecologist, I have listed a few go-to responses for you to use when facing a difficult situation in college. Some sentences are from college-age patients. These suggestions are listed in Chapter 1, however I think they are worth repeating:

- "No, I can't leave the party with you. I'm staying with my friends."
- "No. I'm not ready for sex."
- "No, I don't want to have sex. I just got my period, and it's really heavy. I need to go home."
- "Eww, what is that bump? I can't have sex with you because you have bumps down there."
- "This party is making me uncomfortable. Let's go!"

Ultimately you should decide for yourself what makes you feel comfortable to say in a difficult or unsafe situation. The most important part is to practice your go-to responses in advance of going to college so you feel confident that you know what to say if a difficult situation arises.

Final Thoughts

- You cannot control anyone else; you can only control yourself.
- You are not responsible for anyone else's actions, but you are absolutely responsible for your own.
- "Sex" includes all forms of expression, not just intercourse. Be aware of what you are choosing to do and what the physical and emotional consequences may be.
- If you decide to have sex, be sure that you are doing it for the right reason, not because you think you're supposed to.
- Remember that your choices about sexuality can affect how you feel about yourself.
- Be sure that the person you choose to have sex with is absolutely worth it. There are millions of people to choose from in the world, so if the one you're with disrespects you or mistreats you, move on.
- Think through your actions first and avoid random sexuality.
- Have your go-to sentences prepared in advance to help you get out of an uncomfortable or unsafe situation.
- Make sure that the choices you make are in keeping with the woman you want to be.

Your decisions about sexuality are very personal and private and only for you to make. No judgment. If you do choose to be sexually active in college, my best advice is this...No quick decisions or random actions. Instead, be prepared!

Think through carefully what actions you will take in advance to be sure that your choices are consistent with your personal values and live up to the standards you've set for yourself. Have your go-to responses ready in case you change your mind. Read and understand the next few chapters on contraception and prevention of sexually transmitted infections so you can protect yourself. This thoughtful approach to your sexuality will help you stay healthy and safe in college and be happy with outcomes of your actions.

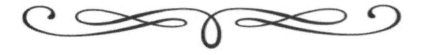

"*Give thought to who you really are*
and
How to make choices that are
consistent with
Your best vision of yourself."

-M. Susan Scanlon, M.D.
The Gyne's Guide

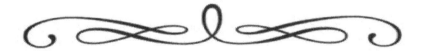

Chapter 14
Condoms and Beyond:
The Do's and Don'ts of Contraception

This chapter covers the different Do's and Don'ts for various forms of contraception that every sexually active college woman should read, understand, and follow.

What is Contraception?

According to the American Congress of OB/GYN: Contraception is a method to deliberately prevent a woman from getting pregnant.

The purpose of this chapter is to provide you with the most comprehensive information presently available about what you can do to prevent unwanted pregnancy while you're in college.

A Gynecologist's Perspective
••••••••••••••••••••••••••••••

Most of my college-age patients think they are invincible and nothing bad will happen to them. Many think it's OK to follow some rules and not others. From my perspective, this random approach is dangerous, especially when it comes to preventing unwanted pregnancy.

My goal is not to tell you what is right or wrong, because that is for you to decide based on your personal values. I encourage you to be responsible, think things through, and make careful decisions.

Every woman regardless of her religious, ethnic or socioeconomic background can get pregnant if she has sex. As a gynecologist, I would recommend that all sexually active people of any background use contraception if they are not prepared to become a parent.

If You Don't Want to Have a Baby in College, then You have Two Choices:
1) Don't have sex.
2) Be organized and use contraception.
If You're Going to Use Contraception, then Be Responsible and Follow Two Rules:
1) Use it properly.
2) Use it every time you have sex.

The contraception information outlined on the following pages is very detailed and may seem intimidating. Don't let the amount of information be overwhelming. Read it through slowly to understand the different forms of contraception available. Being prepared is an important part of responsible adulthood. If you decide to be sexually active in college, use this guide to help you decide how to best take care of yourself. Then talk to your doctor about your choices.

Abstinence

- Abstinence is defined as the voluntary action of not having sex.
- If you want to be certain that you will not become pregnant in college, abstinence is your best strategy.
- The failure rate is 0%

Do's
1. Pick this form of contraception if you want a guarantee that you will not get pregnant.
2. Select this option to improve your odds of avoiding an STD.

Don'ts
1. Do not fall for the argument that you are abstaining if the guy does not ejaculate inside your vagina. Abstinence does not equal "pulling out." You can get pregnant if you choose any form of contraception other than abstinence.

Condoms

- Condoms are a barrier form of contraception that block the sperm from getting into the vagina and reaching the cervix.

- Male condoms are made of latex (a type of rubber) or polyurethane (a type of plastic) and are lubricated or non-lubricated. There are also "natural" male condoms made of lambskin, but these are not as effective as latex or polyurethane condoms to prevent STDs, including HIV.
- The lubricant on the outside of a male condom, Nonoxynol-9, is a spermicide that helps kill sperm that may have gotten into your vagina.
- Female condoms are made of nitrile and have a silicone lubricant on the inside.
- The Failure Rate of a properly used male latex condom is typically 18%. The failure rate of a properly used female condom is 21%. Condoms have high failure rates because they can break or fall off and therefore should be used in addition to another form of contraception.
- Condoms have the added benefit in also helping to reduce the transmission of sexually transmitted diseases.

Do's

1. Use a condom every time you have sex.
2. Have a condom in your purse. You should never rely on anyone else for your protection.
3. Pick a condom brand that is effective and comfortable for your vagina. Latex condoms are the best. If you are sensitive or allergic to latex, pick one made of polyurethane. If the Nonoxynol-9 on the lubricated condom causes irritation, try a non-lubricated condom instead. When extra moisture is needed, always use a water-based lubricant, such as Astroglide, when using a male condom.
4. Consider a female condom if you prefer to be completely in charge of the use of a condom. Insert it up to eight hours before sex initiates. You can use either a water-based or oil-based lubricant with a female condom.
5. Store condoms in a cool dry place so they don't dry out and crack. Be sure to check the expiration date on the condom box because expired condoms can break easily.
6. For oral sex, a male condom is recommended to prevent STDs in your mouth. There are flavored brands available.
7. For anal intercourse (often painful; not a common activity with

my patients), a non-lubricated male condom is recommended. The Nonoxynol-9 on a lubricated condom increases the risk of transmission of STDs and HIV, which is increased with anal intercourse. Avoid female condoms because they cannot be inserted properly in the anus. Use a water-based lubricant to reduce pain and rectal tears.

8. If the condom falls off or the female condoms falls out, go to the student health service for an STD screen and start Plan B to prevent pregnancy. (See the section on Plan B for emergency contraception.)

9. Understand How to Properly Use a Male Condom
   - Carefully remove the condom from the package. Do not use your teeth, nails or anything else that may be sharp because you can damage the condom.
   - Leave the condom rolled until it is put on a hard penis.
   - If the condom is put on inside out, throw it out and open a new one.
   - Allow the tip of the condom some room above the tip of the penis (the reservoir).
   - Squeeze the tip of the condom (the reservoir) to let out the air, and then start to roll the condom down the shaft of the penis.
   - Check to be sure that the condom does not look broken and that there is space at the tip. This space (the reservoir) is to catch the semen before and during ejaculation.
   - With the condom on properly, insert the penis for intercourse.
   - After ejaculation, hold the base of the condom firmly in place when removing the penis from the vagina. This should be done before the penis becomes soft to prevent the condom from coming off inside the vagina.
   - Pull the condom off without spilling the fluid, and throw the condom in the trash.
   - If you need a diagram, refer to the website: http://www.health.ny.gov/publications/instructions_male_condom.pdf

10. Understand How to Properly Use a Female Condom
    - Carefully remove the condom from the package so you don't damage it.
    - You can insert it up to eight hours before intercourse.

- Identify the inner (larger) ring and the outer (smaller) ring.
- Rub the condom gently to distribute the inner lubricant.
- Press the sides of the larger inner ring together with your thumb and middle finger to make the shape of a skinny oval, and then insert the ring into the vagina like a tampon. You may have to squat or lie down to be able to insert it.
- Push the larger inner ring up high into the vagina and around the cervix. The vagina is not an endless tube; it ends in the cervix, which you will feel if you reach high enough (about the length of your index or middle finger).
- Make sure that the condom does not get twisted.
- The smaller outer ring should be positioned at the opening of your vagina.
- For intercourse, put a few drops of water-based lubricant at the opening of the condom or on the penis. Gently guide the penis into the condom. An oil-based lubricant is also ok with the female condom.
- If there is stickiness, rubbing or a sound, add more lubricant.
- After intercourse, twist the outer ring before pulling the condom out so that the semen is trapped inside the condom. Then gently pull the condom out of the vagina and throw it away in the trash.
- Practice inserting a female condom a few times before you want to use it for contraception. Practice is helpful and will give you more confidence to actually use it.
- If you need a diagram, refer to the website: http://www.health.ny.gov/publications/9571.pdf

Don'ts

1. Do not "forget" to put on the condom. Be responsible, take care of yourself, and use a condom every time you have sex.
2. Don't fall for the arguments that "It doesn't feel good" or "You don't need a condom if you're on the pill." These arguments do not have your best interests in mind. If the guy refuses to put on the condom, then don't have sex, and break up with the guy.
3. If you have skin sensitivities, don't use fancy condoms with different tastes, smells, types that heat up or have ribs. Frequently women who feel burning after sex are just sensitive to the type of condom being selected or the Nonoxynol-9 in the lubricant. Sometimes guys think women will like these added

features, but oftentimes, their vaginas do not.

4. Do not use a condom that looks like it has an irregular color, feels dried out, looks cracked or old or feels sticky. It could break.
5. Do not use a male and female condom at the same time.
6. Do not rinse out and re-use condoms. They are not effective the second time. They're inexpensive, so buy a new one.
7. Don't throw a used condom into the toilet. It will clog the toilet.

Important Research to Understand

Results of the Contraceptive CHOICE Project were published in November 2013 and concluded that intrauterine devices and contraceptive implants have the highest rates of continuation of use by women between ages 14 and 45.

In other words, more women were satisfied with IUDs and contraceptive implants than OCPs, vaginal rings or contraceptive patches, and therefore they kept using the contraception.

This is important because consistent use of contraception is the best way to prevent pregnancy. According to researchers, "These long acting reversible forms of contraception (IUDs and contraceptive implants) are more than 20-fold more effective at preventing unintended pregnancy than the commonly used OCP, vaginal ring, or patch."

The bottom line is that the research recommends that the first choice of contraception should be an IUD or contraceptive implant. If one of these two forms of contraception is medically not appropriate for you or has intolerable side effects, then the second choice would be OCPs, vaginal rings, hormone injections or contraceptive patches.

Talk to your doctor about this study and what contraceptive option is best for you.

Intrauterine Devices

- An IUD is a convenient, long-acting, form of contraception that is well liked by my patients. It works by changing the way sperm move (hinders sperm), thickening the cervical mucus (blocks the sperm), creating inflammation inside the uterine cavity (kills the sperm), and thinning the lining of the uterus.

- A copper IUD is the most effective form of emergency contraception. In addition to the above forms of action, it may also work by the prevention of implantation of a fertilized egg.
- Most patients tolerate the insertion very well, experiencing only a temporary cramping feeling for a few minutes up to one or two days. Your doctor will insert the small T-shaped flexible device through the opening in your cervix and into your uterine cavity without making any incisions.
- It is possible that the IUD will not fit into your uterus if you have not had a baby yet because the size of your uterine cavity may be too small. Your doctor will measure you to see if it will fit.
- There are two strings attached to the IUD that can be felt in the top of your vagina. These strings help you to know that the IUD remains in place. However, you and your partner will typically not feel the strings during intercourse. The doctor will use these strings to remove or replace the IUD.
- There are two types of IUDs available in the U.S. in 2016:
  - Hormonal IUDs: Mirena (lasts five years), Skyla (lasts three years) and Liletta (lasts three years)
  - Copper (non-hormonal) IUD: Paragard (lasts 10 years)
- The Failure Rate of an IUD:
  - Mirena and Liletta: Less than 1% (0.2%)
  - Skyla: Less than 1% (0.9%)
  - Paragard: Less than 1% (0.8%)

Do's

1. Consider an IUD if you want a hassle-free, long-term form of contraception. This option is very effective, and there's nothing for you to do for several years after the insertion.
2. If you have heavy periods, the hormonal IUD Mirena, would be a great option because it provides contraception with the added benefit of making your periods lighter. Paragard does not have this benefit.
3. Check the strings once per month to be sure that the IUD has not fallen out or shifted. The expulsion rate is 3-6%
4. Return to the doctor's office 4-6 weeks after the IUD insertion to confirm that the IUD is sitting properly in your uterus.

5. Call the doctor if you are having any problems with the IUD such as pain, fever, heavy vaginal discharge or abnormal periods.
6. Understand the risks of an IUD. These risks are not common:
    - Women who get pregnant with an IUD in place have an increased risk that the pregnancy will be in the fallopian tube (ectopic pregnancy) compared to other forms of contraception. An ectopic pregnancy is a high-risk condition. If you do not get your period and have an IUD in place, check a pregnancy test. See your doctor if you experience pain in your pelvis or think that you could be pregnant.
    - There is a rare risk that the IUD will push through the wall of the uterus, called a perforation. The warning signs would include pain and abnormal bleeding. Call your doctor's office or school health service if you have these symptoms.
    - Exposure to an STD while an IUD is in place can lead to a severe pelvic infection, called pelvic inflammatory disease and infertility (inability to have a baby).
7. Understand any religious implications. The copper IUD may possibly work by preventing the implantation of a fertilized egg. If your religious beliefs are in conflict with this fact, then this option of contraception may not be for you.

Don'ts
1. Do not select this form of contraception if you refuse to use a condom because of the risk of exposure to an STD, which can progress to a severe pelvic infection (PID) and infertility.
2. Do not have an IUD inserted if you are pregnant, have an undiagnosed cause of abnormal uterine bleeding, a history of some forms of cancer, recent PID, or if your uterus has an abnormal shape. Discuss your medical history with your doctor to decide if an IUD is appropriate for you.
3. You may not want a hormonal IUD if you already have light periods because the flow usually becomes even lighter and may stop all together. In addition, spotting between periods can become a problem for patients with a hormonal IUD.
4. You may not want the copper IUD inserted if your periods are already heavy or painful because often the period becomes heavier with more cramps once this type of IUD is inserted.

- A contraceptive implant contains a low dose of the hormone called progesterone and prevents pregnancy by preventing ovulation, thickening the cervical mucus (blocking the sperm) and thinning the lining on the inside of the uterus.
- It is a small, painless matchstick-sized device inserted under the skin of the upper arm. It is not usually noticeable to anyone else when they look at your arm.
- This form of contraception is very convenient, lasts three years, and is well liked by many young patients.
- The insertion is well tolerated by most patients, done in the doctor's office or college health service, and requires only a local anesthetic. The insertion requires a tiny incision.
- Nexplanon is the only FDA-approved contraceptive implant in the U.S. at the time of this publication. It is the same medication as Implanon. (The company changed the name to Nexplanon due to the new design for safer implant insertion.)
- The Failure Rate of the Contraceptive Implant: Less than 1% (0.05%)

Do's
1. Consider this option if you want an estrogen-free, reliable, long-term form of contraception.
2. Check your arm occasionally to be sure that you still feel the implant. Call the doctor if you can't feel it in your arm because it may have shifted locations. Talk to the doctor if you have pain.

Don'ts
1. Do not use an implant if you have an allergy or reactions to progesterone products, barium sulfate (which makes the implant visible on an x-ray) or magnesium stearate.
2. If you have a Body Mass Index (BMI) above 27.2, do not use Nexplanon because it may not be effective for contraception due to your weight. Refer to the BMI chart in Chapter 3.
3. If you have irregular periods, this may not be the best choice for you because some patients with an implant complain of abnormal periods.

- Combination OCPs contain synthetic estrogen and progesterone hormones that work by suppressing ovulation, thickening the cervical mucus (blocks the sperm), and thinning the lining on the inside of the uterus. There are approximately 40 different brands of OCPs for your doctor to choose from to find one that's right for you.
- Progesterone-only OCPs, often called the "mini-pill" have only one hormone, progesterone, and work in a similar way as combination pills. This may be a good choice if you cannot take estrogen or have worsening migraines on combination OCPs.
- The Failure Rate: Less than 1% (0.1%) when the pills are taken perfectly (same time every day, no missed pills). The actual failure rate for OCPs is 9 percent during the first year, due primarily to missed pills or forgetting to restart the pill on time.

Do's

1. Pick a realistic time of the day to take your pill. First thing in the morning may not work if you sleep later on the weekends. Before bed is probably not the best because your nighttime schedule may vary with school and social activities. My patients tell me that 6 or 7 o'clock at night seems to work the best.
2. Take the pill at the same time every day. Set your cell phone alarm to keep you on schedule. If you vary the time you take the pill by more than 24 hours apart, you can have vaginal bleeding between periods, and you increase your risk of getting pregnant.
3. Understand that the first four pills of the pack are very important pills to take on time because they prevent the recruitment of an egg. This is critical to prevent ovulation and therefore prevent pregnancy.
4. If you miss one pill, take it as soon as you remember. You can take the missed pill and the next pill at the same time. If you miss two pills in a row in the first two weeks, then take the two missed tablets, then two more tablets the next day, followed by one tablet daily for the remainder of the pack. However, in this situation, the pack is no longer effective for contraception, and you will need an additional form of contraception (a back-up plan). Try your best to remember to take your pills on time.

5. Always finish a pack that you have started. To change brands or to stop OCPs and switch to a new form of contraception, always finish your pack. If you quit in the middle, you will start bleeding, which makes it confusing about when to start the new brand.
6. Always use a condom in addition to the OCP to prevent STDs.
7. Notify your doctor if you have abnormal periods; headaches; pelvic, chest or leg pain; leg swelling; shortness of breath; or visual changes while taking OCPs.
8. According to Mayo Clinic, some meds decrease the effectiveness of OCPs, including ampicillin, tetracycline, penicillin V, Norvir, barbiturates, Fulvicin, Rifampin, troglitazone, and seizure meds.
9. Call your doctor if you have missed pills or have any questions.

Don'ts

1. Do not take OCPs if you have had a blood clot in your legs, lungs, or eyes; prior stroke or heart attack; Factor V Leiden (clotting disorder); migraines with aura (visual changes); uncontrolled diabetes or hypertension; gallbladder or liver problems; active pregnancy; a history of breast, uterine or ovarian cancer; or take other female hormone medications. Always be sure to review your past medical history and your family history with your doctor before starting OCPs.
2. Do not call your doctor at 11 o'clock at night on Sunday because you just realized that you forgot to call for a refill of your pills. Instead, when you pick up your last pill pack from the pharmacy, call the doctor for a refill. Be organized and respectful of others by calling during office hours with adequate time for the staff to review your chart and confirm the medical information needed for the doctor to refill any medication.
3. Don't quit in the middle of a pack. It will cause abnormal bleeding.
4. Do not rely on the OCP for contraception if you have had two episodes of missing pills in one pack because you can get pregnant. Finish the pack, but be aware that you will need to use a back-up form of contraception like condoms, spermicide, or abstinence until you get your next period.
5. Don't give your unused OCP packs to a friend. You don't know if she has a medical condition that would make it unsafe for her to take the medication. Instead, refer your friend to her doctor. Save your unused packs in case you restart the OCP.

Caution about Blood Clots on OCPs

Be aware that the biggest risk of OCP medications is a blood clot in the blood vessels of the legs, lungs, heart, eyes or brain. Although this potential risk is uncommon, it is harmful and sometimes deadly. It is important that you understand the symptoms of a blood clot so you know when to call the doctor. In addition, review the scenarios that can increase the risk of a clot so that you can stop the pill if these circumstances arise.

Symptoms of a Blood Clot on OCPs
- Chest pain, chest pressure, shortness of breath, leg pain, leg swelling, redness or heat in the leg, visual changes, worst headache of your life, seizures or loss of consciousness
- If you have any of these symptoms, call the doctor immediately. Let the doctor know your symptoms and that you are taking OCPs.

Scenarios that Increase your Risk of a Blood Clot on OCPs
    Stop your OCP if any of the following happens:
- Trauma or major car accident (not a fender bender) that necessitates prolonged bed rest or hospitalization for an extended period of time.
- Major surgery (a major procedure, not having your wisdom teeth out) necessitates stopping your OCP the week prior to surgery; resume the pill once you are healed and fully ambulatory. Ask your surgeon about it.
- Having a cast or boot put onto your arm or leg due to an orthopedic injury—this leads to immobilization of the arm or leg, and is the most common time I see patients with a blood clot on OCPs.

Vaginal Ring and Contraceptive Patch

- These options work similarly to OCPs but are topical, not oral. The ring is inserted into the vagina; the patch is applied to the skin of the arm. Both release synthetic estrogen and progesterone into the blood stream to provide contraception.
- These convenient methods of contraception have the benefits of an OCP without having to remember to take a pill every day.

- The only FDA-approved vaginal ring available in the U.S. in 2015 was Nuvaring. The contraceptive patch was Ortho-Evra.
- The ring needs to be stored in the refrigerator until it's ready for use. Once inserted into your vagina, the heat from your body activates the ring.
- You will be exposed to a 60% greater amount of estrogen if you use the patch than if you use a low dose OCP, which may increase clotting. Ask your doctor if this option is safe for you.
- The Failure Rate of each of these options is 9%.

Do's

1. Consider these options of contraception if you like OCPs but can't remember to take them every day.
2. Tell your doctor if you have a family history of clotting or stroke.
3. Use these properly: Insert the vaginal ring into the vagina or apply the patch to your arm. Keep the ring inside the vagina/patch on arm continuously for three weeks. Remove the ring/patch on the first day of the fourth week to have a period. Reinsert a new ring/apply a new patch exactly seven days after you removed it to begin the same timed schedule again.
4. Set your cell phone alarm to keep you on schedule.
5. If the patch falls off, reapply. If the ring falls out, immediately rinse it off and reinsert it. If the ring is reinserted into the vagina *within three hours*, it is still effective for contraception.

Don'ts

1. Do not rely on a vaginal ring for contraception if you discover that it has fallen out for more than three hours. The ring is dependent on body temperature to be effective, so if you realize it has been out for more than three hours, you need to insert another ring. If you don't have one, then abstain from sex and call your doctor.
2. Rifampin and anti-seizure meds may make the ring less effective.
3. If you weigh more than 198 pounds, the patch may not be effective.

Long-Acting Progesterone Injection

- Frequently referred to as "The Shot," this hormonal form of contraception contains synthetic progesterone and works by preventing ovulation, thickening the cervical mucus (blocks the sperm) and thinning the lining of the uterus.

- The contraceptive injection available in the U.S. in 2016 is Depo-Medroxyprogesterone Acetate or DMPA (Depo-Provera).
- DMPA is injected into a muscle of the buttock or upper arm once every three months. A subcutaneous form is also available for injection under the skin.
- The Failure Rate: Less than 1%, if the injection is given on time. The actual failure rate is approximately 6% due to variation in the injection schedule.

Do's

1. Consider this option if you can't remember to use other forms of contraception consistently. The medication lasts three months, so you would have the convenience of only four shots per year.
2. Be sure to get the first injection within the first seven days of your period to prevent pregnancy immediately.
3. Many doctors recommend this option if a patient has had a prior unplanned pregnancy and is not good at taking pills or using other forms of contraception.
4. If you are not able to take estrogen or have a seizure disorder, DMPA may be a good choice for contraception.

Don'ts

1. Beware of this option if you have depression or migraines. I find my patients who have these medical conditions can have a worsening of their mood and headaches when they use DMPA.
2. 50% of women will stop having a menstrual flow one year after using this medication. If this will bother you, choose a different option.
3. Be aware of the increased risk of weight gain reported by many patients who use this product (approximately five pounds).
4. Do not use this medication for a prolonged period of time because of the possible risk of thinning of the bones. Talk to your doctor about the longest amount of time that it is safe for you to use this medication.
5. If you want to get pregnant soon, DMPA is not the best choice of contraception for you because it can take nine to 18 months to wear off and for ovulation to begin again.

- Each of these barrier methods of contraception blocks the sperm from getting to the cervix. My patients do not commonly use these forms of contraception due to the high failure rate and the mess of the spermicide.
- The diaphragm looks like a shallow flexible cup with a wide rim; the cervical cap looks like a thimble.
- Spermicide is necessary.
- The Failure Rate of a diaphragm or cervical cap is 12%.

Do's

1. Consider one of these barrier methods if you want to avoid all forms of hormonal contraception and do not want a long-acting contraceptive.

Don'ts

1. Do not use this form of contraception if you have sensitivity to Nonoxynol-9.
2. Do not choose this as your contraceptive method if you know that you will not be good at remembering to insert the device before intercourse. Many college women have the best intentions, but get pregnant because of inconsistent use of contraception. If you're not good at remembering things, choose another form of contraception.

┌───┐
│   **Withdrawal**   │
└───┘

- Withdrawal is having the male partner "pull out" of your vagina before ejaculation.
- Warning: There is always pre-ejaculation semen that is released, which contains enough sperm to get you pregnant.
- The Failure Rate for withdrawal is 22%. This is a very high risk for a woman who does not want to have a baby in college. It means you could possibly get pregnant about once in every four times you have intercourse if you use withdrawal as your only contraception. Think this through carefully and discuss this with your partner. I'd recommend that you choose a safer form of contraception.

Natural Family Planning

- This form of contraception relies on the ability to time ovulation. Abstinence from intercourse is required on the days surrounding ovulation in order to prevent pregnancy.
- This option is for women who prefer an "all-natural" approach and those with certain religious beliefs.
- It requires a regular predictable menstrual cycle in order to calculate your fertile days. Do not have intercourse on the fertile days.
- If you have irregular periods, this is not a good choice for contraception because your ovulation will not be predictable.
- Use an app to help you calculate when you are fertile, such as Clue period tracker.
- The Failure Rate for Natural Family Planning is 24%. This is a high failure rate because there is not a perfect way to predict ovulation. If you absolutely do not want to get pregnant, or if your periods are not regular, this is not a good choice for contraception.

Emergency Contraception

- This is exactly as it says: an emergency form of contraception.
- There are two approaches: Take Plan B One-Step or have a copper IUD inserted by the doctor (see IUDs above for info).
- Plan B One-Step, called "the morning after pill" or "post-coital contraception," is available at the pharmacy without a prescription.
  - It works by preventing ovulation, interfering with fertilization of an egg, or preventing the implantation of a fertilized egg.
  - It will not cause a fertilized egg that has already implanted into your uterus to miscarry or abort. If you are already pregnant when you take it, this method will not work.
  - Plan B One-Step will reduce the risk of pregnancy by 95% if you take it within 48 hours of unprotected intercourse, and 89% if you take it within 72 hours of unprotected intercourse.

Do's

1. Have a copper IUD inserted or start Plan B as an emergency treatment if you had unprotected intercourse or if your contraceptive method has failed. Examples include: if you didn't use a condom; found the condom broke or fell off; forgot to take your OCPs; the vaginal ring fell out during sex and you realized it three days later and didn't reinsert the ring; the patch fell off and you didn't reapply; or the IUD fell out.
2. Start Plan B One-Step as soon as possible, ideally within 48 hours. It can be taken up to five days after unprotected intercourse, but its effectiveness decreases the longer you wait to take it after having sex.
3. If you are a victim of sexual assault, get help right away. Call the police, go to the hospital, and start Plan B One-Step as soon as possible.

Don'ts

1. Don't use Plan B as your only contraceptive method of choice. Some college women choose to just use Plan B whenever they have sex rather than having a regular contraceptive method. This is an unwise approach to your health. Instead, Plan B One-Step is intended for occasional use in the event of a problem with your usual contraceptive method or in the case of sexual assault.

Note: Copper IUDs and Plan B One-Step have the possible action of interfering with the implantation of a fertilized egg. If this is in conflict with your religious beliefs, talk to your doctor about your concerns and options.

Final Thoughts

I realize that this is a heavy chapter, and the information can be overwhelming. If you have more questions, talk to your doctor or the student health service. The best advice I can give you about contraception is to be prepared. If you don't want to have a baby in college, either don't have sex or use contraception consistently and properly every time. No excuses! Plan for your contraception as wisely as you plan for your future.

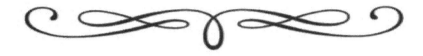

*"Commitment means
staying loyal to what you said
you were going to do long after the
mood you said it in has left you."*

-Unknown

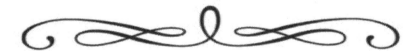

Chapter 15
Avoiding Sexually Transmitted Diseases

Casey

Casey came into the office for an evaluation of a "bump" on the outside of her vagina. She stated she was a virgin. Casey said she had a boyfriend but wanted to wait to have sex until she knew that she had found the right person. On exam she had herpes. Casey was upset and confused and denied having sex with anyone. After further questioning, she revealed that she had oral sex with her boyfriend, Tim. She said she knew that Tim had cold sores, but that he did not have genital herpes. Casey did not realize that oral cold sores were herpes and could be transmitted to the genitalia through oral sex. Casey said she felt devastated when she learned that the bump near her vagina was herpes.

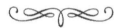

Olivia

Olivia made an appointment in my office because she developed a vaginal discharge two months after starting her freshman year. When she first got to school, Olivia had a light class schedule and a lot of time on her hands. She didn't know anyone at her new college, so she started hanging out every day with a guy from her dorm named Matt. Although she had only one boyfriend in high school and had taken a long time before doing anything other than kissing, things progressed quickly, and she started to have sex with Matt. She was not experienced with contraception and relied on her new boyfriend to provide the protection. Matt said he didn't like to use condoms because "they don't feel good." He assured Olivia that he didn't have any STDs, and that he would "pull out" for contraception. Soon after they began having intercourse, Olivia found out that Matt was cheating on her with his old girlfriend. Since then, she had a "weird, smelly discharge" and vaginal itching. Olivia came into the office for STD testing and was diagnosed with trichomoniasis. Olivia felt very upset that Matt cheated on her and gave her an STD. Furthermore, she recognized that she typically would not have had sex so quickly with a guy, especially unprotected sex. Olivia said that she felt bad about the sexual choices she was making in college and knew that she needed to make some changes.

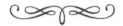

Stephanie

Stephanie scheduled a routine check-up over Thanksgiving break. She said she was doing well in school and had a nice boyfriend named Kurt. When her STD screening test results returned positive for chlamydia, Stephanie was very upset. She was in an exclusive relationship and confused about how she could have gotten an STD. Back at school, she confronted Kurt, who finally admitted that he cheated on her but that "it only happened once." Kurt explained to Stephanie that he really did love her, but he had gotten drunk, had sex with a girl he didn't know and didn't want to tell her because "it was a stupid mistake." Because Stephanie didn't know at the time about what had happened, she continued to have sex as before, without a condom, because she believed they were exclusive. Kurt infected Stephanie with chlamydia after cheating with an unknown girl. Getting an STD, especially while in an "exclusive" relationship, made Stephanie feel deceived, sad, and angry.

A Gynecologist's Perspective

I've heard similar stories to these hundreds of times during 19 years in the office. Sexually transmitted diseases are a common problem in college, so be aware of what you are choosing to do, the physical and emotional consequences of your actions, and **always** use a condom.

Cheating is a frequent occurrence in college relationships. Both Olivia and Stephanie were exposed to an STD due to their partners cheating, and the experience was very difficult to handle. Perhaps Kurt does love Stephanie, but they're in college and many people, including Kurt, are experimenting and making mistakes.

Unfortunately, mistakes can lead to a sexually transmitted disease. It's certainly not these women's fault for getting an STD, and the responsibility lies with Matt and Kurt. However, condoms could protect these women better in the future.

Casey was also devastated about getting exposed to an STD because she didn't know about getting herpes from oral sex. In the future, she could protect herself by abstaining from sex when Tim has a cold sore.

Dating is a fun part of college, and you may choose to date many different people to find a meaningful relationship. However, as addressed in the sexuality chapter, you don't have to have sex just because you date. I encourage you to be cautious with your sexuality to reduce your probability of exposure to an STD and the emotional havoc that follows the diagnosis.

Your only guarantee of avoiding an STD is to abstain from sex. If you do choose to have sex, a monogamous relationship is the best approach because the statistics indicate that the more sexual partners you have, the higher probability you will get an STD. You'd hate to meet the person of your dreams some day and then find out you're infertile because someone in college infected you with an STD, especially if you don't even remember who that someone was.

Every year, I have patients with experiences like Casey, Olivia, and Stephanie. None of them expected to be exposed to an STD in college, and each felt bad about what had happened. The important point from these stories is this: Whether you are in a committed, exclusive relationship or experimenting with multiple partners, you need protection every time you have sex. Whether it's oral, anal or vaginal intercourse, having sex exposes you to the risk of STDs, so protect yourself. If your partner won't put the condom on then ask yourself, "Is this really the right partner for me?" If he can't respect your right to protection, don't have sex with him and think about getting a new partner!

- STDs are common: there are millions of new cases reported every year in the United States and worldwide.
- 13% of college women will be exposed to an STD.
- Anyone who has contact by vaginal, oral or anal sex can get exposed to an STD. Contact with the skin, genitals, mouth, rectum or body fluids of another person with an STD puts you at risk.
- People with an STD do not always have noticeable symptoms and can pass it on to another person without even knowing it.
- Hopefully, if someone knows they have an STD, he or she will get treatment and tell all partners about it *before* having sex.
- Various bacteria and viruses cause STDs; antibiotics treat the bacteria, but there is no cure for many of the viruses.
- A primary risk factor for getting an STD is having multiple partners in your lifetime. In addition, if your partner has had multiple partners in his/her lifetime, you are at increased risk for getting an STD.
- Use of intravenous drugs, or if your partner uses IV drugs, puts you at serious risk of STDs, especially HIV and hepatitis.
- Sexual acts that tear or break the skin allow easier transmission of STDs, especially herpes and HIV. Even small cuts that do not bleed allow bacteria to pass back and forth.
- There is a common myth that oral sex does not put someone at risk of getting a sexually transmitted infection: this is not true. Oral sex puts you at risk of getting herpes, HPV, gonorrhea, chlamydia, syphilis, and HIV.
- Condoms and dental dams can reduce the risk of transmission of STDs with oral sex. Information on dental dams is detailed later in this chapter. Condoms are discussed in Chapter 14.
- Anal sex carries a high risk of transmission of STDs because the rectal tissue is fragile and can tear easily. Body fluids that carry the sexually transmitted bacteria and viruses are exposed to those small rectal cuts and pass on the STD.
- All sexually active women up to age 25 should have STD screening every year because STDs are most common between ages 13 and 25. Starting at age 26, your doctor will discuss your risk factors and recommend when STD screening is appropriate.

Human Papilloma Virus

- Human Papilloma Virus is the *most common* STD. 80% of people will be exposed to this virus in their lifetime.
- Typically HPV is a temporary problem: 95% of young people will clear the virus from their body within two to four years.
- HPV is spread by skin-to-skin contact. You do not have to have sexual intercourse to spread HPV. The female condom may protect you better from the virus than the male condom because it can cover more genital skin.
- HPV can cause abnormal pap smears, genital warts and cancer.
- Approximately 15 different strains (types) of HPV are linked to cancer of the cervix, vulva, vagina, anus and penis. These types are known as "high-risk strains." HPV 16 and 18 are the two types with the highest risk of cervical cancer.
- 98% of cervical cancers are associated with HPV.
- 70-82% of cervical cancers are due to High Risk HPV types 16 and 18.
- 25% of women with type 16 will develop cervical cancer.
- 18% of women with type 18 will develop cervical cancer.
- Approximately 12 strains of HPV cause genital warts. These growths may appear on the outside or inside of the vagina, the cervix or on the penis and can spread to nearby skin, the vulva or anus. They look like cauliflower or small skin tags.
- There is an HPV vaccine to prevent several strains of the HPV virus. It is recommended for women and men to receive the vaccine between ages 9 and 26. It is given as a series of injections over several months. I encourage the majority of my patients to get the HPV vaccine to reduce their risk of infection with some of the strains of HPV. Talk to your doctor to see if this vaccine is appropriate for you.

Chlamydia

- Chlamydia is the most commonly *reported* STD in the U.S., and one of the most frequent STDs that I find in my college patients.
- This STD has very few symptoms, which is why it is so common.
- If untreated, chlamydia (a bacteria) can lead to chronic pelvic pain, fallopian tube scarring, tubal pregnancies, and infertility.

Gonorrhea

- Gonorrhea (a bacteria) causes infections in the genitals, rectum, and throat. It's a common infection, especially in sexually active people between 15 and 25 years old.
- The symptoms are typically very mild and confused for the symptoms of a bladder or vaginal infection.
- Getting tested every year is important because an untreated infection causes scarring of the fallopian tubes, infertility, tubal pregnancies, and chronic pelvic pain.

Trichomoniasis

- This STD is very common: 3.7 million people have the infection. It is more common in women than in men.
- Only about 30% of people with trichomoniasis develop any symptoms, so most men and women do not know they carry the STD. The infection is caused by a parasite and transmitted back and forth between vagina and penis. It does not commonly infect the mouth or anus.
- About one in five people get re-infected within three months of treatment. This is most likely from re-exposure from an infected partner or having sex before all the symptoms have gone away (usually seven days). If your symptoms persist or come back, you need to be retested. Be sure your partner is treated and tested before you have sex with him/her again to minimize your risk of re-exposure and re-infection with trichomoniasis.

Herpes

- Herpes is a highly contagious virus that persists throughout your lifetime once you have been exposed.
- The herpes virus causes blisters on the mouth and genitals. The blisters burst, create a crater, crust over and eventually heal.
- The initial symptoms of a herpes infection, called the prodrome, are a stinging, tingling, and "pins-and-needles" sensation. Blisters soon follow.
- Herpes is very contagious anytime during the prodrome and while the blisters and craters are present. Once *all* the craters crust over, the virus is no longer contagious.
- Some people have only one initial viral outbreak, while others have several outbreaks each year. The best way to reduce the

frequency of outbreaks is to keep your immune system strong with plenty of rest, not smoking, and having a healthy lifestyle.

- Herpes can be transmitted to the genitals or mouth by having sex vaginally, anally or orally with a partner who has genital herpes, a cold sore or a "canker sore."
- It can also be spread from one part of your own body to another by touching the blister or crater and then touching another area such as your mouth or eyes. Always wash your hands after touching the oral cold sore or the genital blister or crater.
- There is not a medicine to remove the virus from your body, but the virus can become "dormant", or not active, for many people.
- Medication can be prescribed to treat "outbreaks" of the herpes blisters and make the symptoms less intense. It's most helpful if the medicine is started as soon as the prodrome begins.
- Patients who have several outbreaks each year can take a daily prescription medication, called suppressive therapy, to reduce the frequency of outbreaks. Talk to your doctor to see if suppressive therapy is appropriate for you.

Syphilis

- Syphilis (a bacteria) causes sores that can be hidden in the mouth or under the foreskin of the penis, so it may not be obvious that a sexual partner has syphilis. Your new partner should have a blood test for syphilis prior to having sex.
- There are three stages of syphilis: early (single/multiple sores); late (rash often on hands or feet); and latent (neurologic problems develop up to 30 years after the initial infection).

Hepatitis

- Hepatitis is a virus. Hepatitis B can be transmitted by exposure to bodily fluids from an infected person during sex or sharing needles for drugs. Sharing toothbrushes or razors contaminated with small amounts of infected blood can also transmit Hepatitis B, so do not share these items with your roommate or partner.
- Hepatitis C is transmitted by direct exposure to infected blood.
- Hepatitis B and C cannot be transmitted by casual contact such as coughing or sneezing, shaking hands or sharing food or drinks.
- There is a vaccine to prevent Hepatitis B. There is no vaccine yet to prevent Hepatitis C. Get a blood test to be screened for both.

HIV

- The human immunodeficiency virus attacks certain parts of the immune system. A person infected with HIV can develop acquired immunodeficiency syndrome and eventually die.
- 18% of the people who have HIV are unaware that they are infected with the virus. This statistic is very concerning and a significant reason why you need to use a latex condom every time you have sex.
- All females between 13 and 64 years old should be tested at least once in their lifetime for HIV and then once per year if they are sexually active, especially if they have risk factors. Risk factors include having more than one sexual partner since last being tested for HIV; intravenous drug use; having sex with someone who has used IV drugs; exchanging sex for money; and having sex with men who have sex with other men.
- If you do not want to be tested for HIV, you have the right to "opt-out," however, it is beneficial to be tested.
- Some types of infected bodily fluid transmit HIV through broken skin. It is not transmitted by casual contact, shaking hands, coughing or sneezing, sharing drinks or food, and cannot be transmitted through intact skin.
- It's often transmitted through anal sex because the skin is so fragile in that area. It is also transmitted vaginally if there are small tears in the vaginal mucosa (skin inside the vagina).
- There is no vaccine yet to prevent HIV and no cure for AIDS.

How Do You Know If You Have an STD?

- HPV (virus): abnormal pap smear/HPV positive; genital warts
- Chlamydia (bacteria): persistent vaginal discharge, often yellow in color; pelvic pain; abnormal periods; urinary frequency; painful urination; blood from the rectum; sore throat
- Gonorrhea (bacteria): most women do not have any symptoms; persistent yellow discharge; painful urination; abnormal periods; rectal bleeding or mucus discharge
- Trichomoniasis (parasite): persistent grey, green or yellow vaginal discharge; foul or fishy odor; burning/swelling of vulva; painful urination; painful intercourse

- Herpes (virus): painful blisters on the genitals, mouth/lips or anus; visible craters; flu–like symptoms; burning sensation on the vulva during urination; swollen lymph nodes in the groin
- Syphilis (bacteria): painless genital sore; rash on hands and feet
- Hepatitis B and C (virus): feeling tired; nausea/vomiting; pain in the abdomen; loss of appetite; yellowing of the skin
- HIV (virus): flu-like symptoms; fever; weight loss; fatigue

How to Protect Yourself from an STD

- Condoms are vital to preventing STDs during vaginal or anal sex, or when giving oral sex to a male partner. Detailed information about male and female condoms is outlined in Chapter 14. The key to STD prevention is to use a condom every time!
- Dental Dams are used as protection from STDs during female oral or anal sex. The dental dam is a rectangular piece of latex that stretches across the vulva and anus to act as a barrier. If you are receiving oral sex from your partner, you can use a dental dam on your vulva and anus to prevent getting exposed to your partner's oral STDs, including oral herpes. If you are giving female oral sex or anal sex, you can stretch the dental dam across your partner's vulva or anus to prevent getting sexually transmitted bacteria and viruses into your mouth. Buy one online or make one by cutting a latex condom into a rectangle.
- Finger Condoms are used to protect your hands from STD exposure if there are little cuts on your fingers. Buy them online.

You've Been Diagnosed with an STD... What Now?

Many of my college-age patients think they don't need to have an STD screen at their routine check-up and then are surprised and disappointed to have a positive result. Although the diagnosis enabled them to get treatment and avoid a more severe pelvic infection, they are still typically very upset.

Having gone through this with so many college women, I have the following advice to help you cope with having an STD:
- Don't beat yourself up! Everyone is human and at risk. Forgive yourself, take better precautions, and move forward.

- Get treated, complete the prescription, and then follow up with your doctor. Knowing the active infection is gone will give you piece of mind.
- Address the STD with your partner. It will allow you to gain an understanding of the "how & why" you got exposed and to express how you feel about it. Although a difficult conversation to have, it will help you decide whether to continue the relationship and will give you a sense of closure.
- Talk to a trusted friend or write in a journal about how the experience made you feel. This will help you heal emotionally.
- Seek professional help if you are still struggling with the STD diagnosis and find that it's affecting your self-esteem, social relationships or performance in school. Talking to a counselor can help you to tackle your negative feelings and rebuild your self-confidence. Counselors are available at Student Health.

Talking to Your Partner about STDs

Before Having Sex: It can be difficult to talk about STDs with other people, especially a new boyfriend. My advice is this: Talk about it! Ask a lot of questions before you choose to have sex with someone. You need to be your own best advocate and take care of yourself. If your partner doesn't want to discuss his sexual history, then ask yourself if this person is really the right partner for you. Ideally, both of you should be screened BEFORE you have sex. If he tests positive for a sexually transmitted disease, you'll have to decide if you'll proceed with the relationship. As I've stated many times, in order to prevent STDs, you need to use a condom every time you have sex.

After You've Been Diagnosed with an STD: I'm frequently asked the question, "Should I tell my partner that I have this STD?" It's an especially common question from patients with herpes. The decision is ultimately up to you. However, I personally feel that all people should be forthcoming with STD information and trust in the relationship. The partner may choose to not be with you anymore, but so be it. It's better than not telling him about the STD and then exposing him to the infection. Just think about how it made you feel when you got an STD from someone who didn't tell you. It's a very difficult conversation, but in my opinion, it's the right thing to do.

Final Thoughts

- If you want to be sexually active and avoid STDs, your best strategy would be to choose a long-term, mutually monogamous relationship with a partner who has been tested and has a negative STD screening result before you have sex.
- You need a latex condom every time you have any form of sex.
- You should never rely on anyone else for your protection; you should have a condom in your purse.
- If he won't put the condom on, don't have sex with him. Think it through: Maybe he's not the right partner for you if he won't respect your need for protection.
- Limit your number of sexual partners. The more partners you have in your lifetime, the more likely you will get an STD.
- Ask your partner about his/her sexual history because it's just as important as your own.
- When your doctor recommends doing an STD test, say "OK."
- If your doctor prescribes a medicine for an STD, be sure to complete the entire prescription. If you don't take all of the pills, the infection will likely continue in you. Your partner needs to be treated for the STD too.
- If you find out your present or prior partner has an STD, see your doctor for an STD test and possible treatment. Ask to see your partner's test results to be assured his infection is gone before having sex with him again.
- Get vaccinated against HPV, if approved by your doctor.
- Anytime you think you might have been exposed to an STD, get tested.

A Gynecologist's Perspective

The topics in this chapter make it critical to think about what's important to you and how you will take care of yourself. Make smart choices rather than taking random actions or just trying to "fit in." If you're going to be sexually active, protect yourself! College can be a lot of fun as you meet new people and develop meaningful relationships, but STDs are abundant in college. Be careful! By thinking through your actions, and protecting yourself from STDs, you will have a safer and happier college experience.

Service to Others

Every year, millions of women and girls throughout the world are infected with sexually transmitted diseases due to inadequate education, prevention, and treatment of infection. According to the World Health Organization, "one crucial element of global maternal and child health that has been sorely neglected is the prevention and treatment of sexually transmitted diseases (STDs)." Access to medication in many underserved countries is terribly inadequate. It's hard to believe that in 2016, people around the world still die from severe infections that result from untreated STDs.

I'd encourage you to become aware and involved in the effort to help women around the world achieve greater access to health care.

<u>Organizations Providing STD Treatment to
Underserved Regions in the World</u>

1. <u>National Center for HIV/AIDS, Viral Hepatitis, STD, and TB Prevention:</u> This organization is part of the Centers for Disease Control, and "aims to create the knowledge, tools, and networks that people and communities need to protect their health—through health promotion, prevention of disease, injury, and disability, and preparedness for health threats." www.cdc.gov

2. <u>The World Bank:</u> The main purpose of this organization is to provide financial and technical assistance to developing countries. Its main goal is to reduce poverty and the negative consequences of poverty. www.worldbank.org

3. <u>World Health Organization:</u> Headquartered in Geneva, this organization provides care to 150 countries with the "primary role to direct and coordinate international health within the United Nations' System." www.who.org

Chapter 16
Alcohol Use: Think it Through

Erin

As a college freshman, Erin started to drink alcohol regularly with her new friends. One Saturday night, Erin and a big group of girls decided to get dressed up and go out for "dollar beers" and dancing at a local bar. Erin only brought $7 with her because the beers were cheap and she had a ride to the bar with her friend.

That night, Erin drank too much and became intoxicated. After dancing for hours and getting dehydrated, she passed out in a booth alongside the dance floor. When she woke up, the bar was closing and her friends were nowhere to be found.

Erin was drunk and needed to get back to her dorm. Her friend with the car did not answer her cell phone or respond to her text. The school shuttle didn't travel that far off campus, and Erin did not have any money left for a taxi since she spent her $7 on beer. She decided that she would walk back alone all the way to school. The bar was in a rough part of town, and she began to encounter some pretty scary people along the walk back to the campus. She felt fearful that something might happen to her, but she didn't have any other way home.

Thankfully, a man in his 20s stopped her on the road, flagged down a cab, and paid the driver for her safe return to campus. He wrote his name and address on a piece of paper and told Erin that she could mail him the money. When she asked him why he was doing this for her, he responded that he had a sister around her age, and he would want someone to help his sister if she were in the same situation.

The next day when Erin woke up, she vaguely remembered what had happened. It was the little piece of paper with the young man's name and address on it that jogged her memory.

In my office the following month, Erin told me about what had happened to her, and expressed gratitude that someone looked out for her when she was drunk and vulnerable. The situation really frightened her, and she decided that she needed to make some changes. Erin realized that she needed to drink less, stay with her group of friends, and always have some money in her pocket. She mailed the $10 back to the guy who helped her.

Gynecologist's Perspective

Erin, a smart, nice girl, like most of my patients, was excited to go to college and gain independence away from home. She had some experience drinking beer in high school, but significantly increased the amount she drank when she got to college. She didn't know her limit, got drunk, and put herself in a dangerous situation.

Erin was naïve and really didn't realize that bad things could happen to her. She was not prepared for the consequences of the actions she was taking. In fact, she had never really thought about the importance of safe drinking habits before that night. Erin, like many freshmen, didn't know the problems she might face in college or how she wanted to handle herself in those situations. Thankfully, Erin was OK in the end, but not every girl gets so lucky. If Erin didn't make some changes in her behavior, and continued to drink heavily, she was bound to get hurt.

Year after year I hear countless stories similar to Erin's, and I find that most of my college-age patient's problems are related to alcohol use. It's not only my patient's drinking, it's also the drinking by all the other students around them.

I have written this guidebook because I understand that underage drinking is common in college, and I want you to have the information you need to be safe. Think about how you can take care of yourself in college. Whether you or someone around you is drinking, YOU are at risk. So, BE PREPARED, and take the time to understand the potential consequences of alcohol use and the steps you can take to socialize in a safe and responsible way.

Important Statistics

- According to the National Institute of Health, "the first six weeks of freshman year is an especially vulnerable time for students. There is heavy drinking and alcohol-related consequences because of 'student expectations and social pressures' at the beginning of the school year."
- Research indicates that more than 80 percent of college students drink alcohol. According to a study in 2008, 40 percent of college students reported binge drinking.
- College women who drink excessively are particularly vulnerable to harm, both emotionally and physically. Examples include injury, unplanned pregnancy, STDs, sexual assault, and depression.

Every year, thousands of college students from across the country have problems due to drinking too much alcohol. Erin is not the only woman to have a rough start in college. Don't let this happen to you!

Potential Consequences of Getting Drunk

If you choose to drink alcohol, be aware of the effects it can have on your life:

- Wake up with a hangover and be unable to study the next day. This can affect your grades.
- Say something stupid to a friend that negatively affects your relationship.
- Make poor decisions that put you at risk of injury.
- Drop your smartphone and crack the glass or lose your phone. Either problem is expensive to fix.
- Lose your purse. Lose your money. Spend all your money. In any of these situations, you're out of money.
- Have unprotected sex. Have random sex. Have sex with a stranger. All put you at risk of STDs and unplanned pregnancy. They may also make you feel bad about yourself.
- Get into a fight. Get beat up. Assault someone else. All harmful.
- Be sexually assaulted. A terrible thing for any person.
- Get arrested for driving under the influence of alcohol.
- Develop a drinking problem. This can affect you the rest of your life.

What are the Possible Medical Problems You Can Have Due to Alcohol?

- Malnutrition from poor absorption of nutrients and unhealthy eating patterns.
- Increased risk of cancer (breast, liver, throat, rectum and esophagus). There is a 41 percent higher risk of breast cancer in women who drink two to five drinks per day.
- Depression and suicide are more common in people who exhibit at-risk drinking.

What is "Binge Drinking"?

- Binge drinking means drinking more than three drinks per occasion.
- The result of binge drinking is a sudden spike in the blood alcohol level.
- Binge drinking can lead to poor judgment and risky behavior.
- Binge drinking causes serious health risks to women in college, including intoxication, alcohol poisoning, and sexual assault.

College is a lot of fun, but you need to be sure to take care of yourself.

Three Steps for Smart and Safe Drinking in College

1. Know Your Limit

2. Plan Ahead of the Party

3. Adopt Safe Drinking Habits

How is a Drink Defined?

"One Drink" equals:

- ☐ A 12-ounce beer
- ☐ A 1.25-ounce shot of 80-proof alcohol
- ☐ A 5-ounce glass of wine
- ☐ A 12-ounce wine cooler

If you are wondering how much you can safely drink, calculate the blood alcohol content (BAC) for different drinks that you might consume in college. Then understand what each blood alcohol level means for your body.

1. Determine Your Blood Alcohol Content to Understand Your Limit

BEFORE you go to college, the best approach for you to understand how much alcohol you can safely consume is to look at a blood alcohol calculator website. Plug in your weight, different numbers of drinks, and different amounts of time for drinking, and the website will tell you the estimated BAC. Often the results will tell you by state if you would surpass the legal driving limit if you consumed a certain number of drinks over time.

One helpful website is the blood alcohol calculator at bloodalcoholcalculator.org/#LinkURL

Example 1: 120-pound woman drinking *over 1 hour*

1 beer or shot	BAC: .021	Not impaired
2 beers or shots	BAC: .059	**Possibly impaired**
3 beers or shots	BAC: .097	**Legally impaired**
4 beers or shots	BAC: .134	Legally impaired
5 beers or shots	BAC: .172	Legally impaired
6 beers or shots	BAC: .210	**Pass out/black out**
7 beers or shots	BAC: .324	**Possible death**

This 120-pound woman who is drinking quickly for one hour has an unsafe blood alcohol level after two drinks. Think about that.

Example 2: Now the same 120-pound woman will have a different blood alcohol content when she spreads her drinks *over three hours*.

1 beer or shot	BAC: .0	Not impaired
2 beers or shots	BAC: .025	Not impaired
3 beers or shots	BAC: .063	**Possibly impaired**
4 beers or shots	BAC: .10	**Legally impaired**
6 beers or shots	BAC: .176	Legally impaired
7 beers or shots	BAC: .214	**Pass out/black out**
10 beers or shots	BAC: .328	**Death possible**

This woman has reached an unsafe blood alcohol level by drinking four drinks over three hours. This is an improvement compared to drinking in one hour, but she's still at risk as she continues to drink.

Be aware, it is riskier for this woman to drink shots compared to beer because of the smaller volume. If she's drinking quickly, the shots' smaller volume will make it more likely she will drink too many, putting her into an unsafe BAC quickly. Beer typically is more filling and difficult to consume rapidly in comparison to shots.

Keep in mind that if she continues to drink more and more beer or shots, even slowly over time, alcohol will accumulate in her body, raise her BAC, and put her at risk for alcohol poisoning.

Many students may be surprised to see these charts. They may already be drinking more than would be considered safe. Further, they may be hanging out with friends who also drink too much, too quickly, and think their alcohol consumption is normal.

If you drink alcohol slowly, avoid consuming multiple drinks in a short amount of time, and stop drinking at your safe limit, you can keep your BAC in a lower range and reduce your risks of intoxication and alcohol poisoning. Be smart... educate yourself about your limit, avoid binge drinking, and choose your friends wisely.

2. Understand Other Factors that Influence your Blood Alcohol Level

- <u>Your liver can only process one drink per hour.</u> If you consume more than one drink per hour, your liver will not be able to keep up, and the alcohol will build up in your blood stream and body. If you take medications that process through your liver, this can slow your liver down. If your liver is not working properly, you will have a higher BAC, increasing the risk of alcohol poisoning.

- <u>Eating food before you go out helps slow down alcohol absorption.</u> Some of my patients who have had problems in college related to alcohol have indicated that they did not eat before going out. When I asked them why, some of the replies have included that it is because they didn't want to spend their money, or it was easier to get drunk, or they didn't want the calories. Come on ladies; let's give that thought. You can bring more money; your goal should not be to get drunk; and having a sandwich before you go out is not that many calories. Be aware that eating food does not mean that you can drink more. In fact, according to Mayo Clinic, food can slow the absorption of alcohol, but it will not prevent alcohol poisoning if you binge drink.

- <u>Water Intake is helpful.</u> Alcohol is a diuretic, which means it will make you urinate more, causing dehydration. This adds to your thirst, which can lead to more alcohol consumption. If you are well hydrated, you will avoid this dangerous mistake. Water helps your liver process the alcohol efficiently to eliminate it from your body. In addition, staying well hydrated can help reduce the risk of a hangover the following morning.

- <u>Body Fat:</u> Women with a higher percentage of body fat will have a higher BAC compared to another woman with a lower amount of body fat. Fat absorbs less water, and alcohol metabolism is related to water content.

3. <u>Review the Alcohol Symptom Chart to Further Understand Your Alcohol Limit</u>

It would be helpful if you could identify the symptoms that you could experience at different blood alcohol levels. Then, you could pace your drinking to avoid the symptoms associated with the higher blood alcohol levels. Review the Symptom Chart on the following page so you know what symptoms you'll feel when you are reaching an unsafe blood alcohol level.

Alcohol Symptom Chart

Symptoms	Blood Alcohol Concentration	Impact
• Some loss of judgment • Relaxation • Slight body warmth • Altered mood • Sense of well being	**.02%**	• Decline in visual functions • Decline in ability to perform two tasks at the same time (divided attention)
• Release of inhibition • Exaggerated behavior • May have loss of small muscle control (e.g., focusing your eyes • Impaired judgment • Usually good feeling • Lowered alertness	**.05%**	• Reduced coordination • Reduced ability to track moving objects
• Muscle coordination becomes poor (e.g., balance, speech, vision, reaction time, and hearing) • Harder to detect danger • Judgment, self-control, reasoning, and memory are impaired	**.08%**	• Poor concentration • Short-term memory loss • Reduced information processing capability (e.g., signal detection, visual search) • Impaired perception
• Clear deterioration of reaction time and control • Slurred speech, poor coordination, and slowed thinking	**.10%**	
• Far less muscle control than normal • Vomiting may occur (unless this level was reached slowly or a person has developed a tolerance for alcohol) • Major loss of balance	**.15%**	• Substantial impairment in necessary visual and auditory information processing

The resources for this chart originated with the National Highway Traffic Safety Administration, the National Institute on Alcohol Abuse and Alcoholism, the American Medical Association, the National Commission Against Drunk Driving, and the Centers for Disease Control.
For symptoms at higher BAC, see the following webwite:
www.webmd.com/mental-health/addiction/blood-alcohol?page=2

If your socializing involves alcohol, being prepared in advance of the party will give you the safest experience in college. Think about how you want to handle different social situations you might encounter before you get there, rather than reacting to what is happening in front of you.

1. Program Your Smartphone
- Input the school shuttle service and a local taxi service into your phone. This way, you can always get home safely, especially if you get separated from your friends.
- If alcohol is involved in any social activity, it is better to take a taxi or shuttle home rather than asking a guy to walk you home…especially if the guy has been drinking.
- Helpful apps: Curb, Easy Taxi, Uber, and Lyft have good reviews.

2. Put Money in your Pocket
- Be sure you have money every time you go out! You never want to be stuck somewhere because you didn't have money to get a ride home.
- If your pants don't have a pocket, and you don't want to carry a purse, buy a cell phone case that has a slot for your money.

3. Eat Food before Going Out
- Eat food, such as a bagel, cheese or a sandwich, within 30 minutes of drinking alcohol. Snack throughout the night.
- Food with protein and carbohydrates will help slow down the absorption of alcohol.
- If you don't eat, you can reach your peak blood alcohol concentration within 30 minutes to two hours. If you eat, you can slow that down to one to six hours, depending on the alcohol you choose.
- Caution: According to Mayo Clinic, eating food will not prevent alcohol poisoning if you are binge drinking.

4. Drink a Full Glass of Water Before Leaving for the Party
- Some people drink more alcohol when they first get to the party because they feel thirsty. If you are well hydrated before the party, you will be able to pace yourself better.

- Drinking plenty of water throughout the night will also decrease your risk of a hangover, which will interfere with your schoolwork and activities the next day.

5. Before You Go Out, Decide What Your Drink Limit will Be
- Review a Blood Alcohol Content website to be certain you know your limit. A good example is www.bloodalcoholcalculator.org.
- Choose to stick to your limit and to avoid binge drinking to stay safe. Encourage your friends to do the same.

6. Review Your Sentences
- Review the sentences that you will use if you find yourself in an uncomfortable or unsafe situation while you are out. These suggestions are in Chapter 1, but I think they're worth repeating.
    o "No!"
    o "No, I can't leave the party with you. I'm staying with my friends. Maybe we could meet up tomorrow after class."
    o "No, I don't want any more alcohol. My stomach hurts."
    o "No, I don't want to do shots. The last time I threw up."
    o "This party makes me uncomfortable. Let's go!"

7. Form a Buddy System
- Agree in advance of the party that no girl stays behind.
- Everyone should pick out a friend to watch over throughout the night. Then agree to leave the party with your buddy.
- Also agree with your buddy that you will take her home if she is getting drunk. She should do the same for you.
- Designate some girls to remain sober each night out; they can help and encourage the buddies to stick to a safe alcohol limit.

8. Pick a Time with your Friends to Come Home from the Party
- The later you stay out, the higher possibility you will drink too much and get drunk. This makes you more vulnerable to poor judgment, bad decisions, and increased problems.
- The later the night becomes, the people around you will be increasingly drunk, thereby increasing your risk of injury or sexual assault.
- Agree with your friends to leave the party if the guys are getting drunk. There is a higher risk to you of sexual assault when a group of people around you becomes intoxicated.

Step 3: Adopt Safe Drinking Habits

1. <u>The number one rule of safe drinking</u>: **Avoid Binge Drinking.**
- Binge drinking is defined as having four or more drinks over a short period of time at one event.
- Drink three or less drinks when you go out.

2. <u>Do Not Pre-Party ("Pre-Game").</u>
- Some kids start to drink while they get ready for the party so they are "feeling good" when they get to the party. Some girls don't want to pay for drinks while they are out, so they binge drink in their dorm rooms before going out. They are already drunk when they get to the party and then continue to drink. Do not get into this dangerous habit.

3. <u>Choose beer over hard alcohol.</u>
- You will get a full feeling from drinking beer and will most likely drink less. The feeling of fullness will make it easier to avoid binge drinking with beer rather than hard alcohol.

4. <u>Avoid drinking shots, especially more than one at one time.</u>
- Shots often lead to getting drunk quicker due to binge drinking. Avoid this risky approach to drinking.

5. <u>Pace yourself by drinking slowly.</u>
- Drink only one drink per hour. Your liver cannot process the alcohol any faster.

6. <u>Monitor how much you drink.</u>
- Keep your plastic beer cups, and stack them into your cup as you have another drink. That way, you will be able to keep track of how many drinks you've had and stick to your limit.

7. <u>Fill up on water throughout the night.</u>
- Have a full glass of water between each drink.

8. <u>Eat food throughout the night.</u>
- Snack frequently to help slow the absorption of alcohol.

9. Calculate your blood alcohol level while you are out
- Use a Blood Alcohol Calculator website after you have had some drinks to understand your blood alcohol level. A higher level is associated with riskier behavior, poorer judgment, and alcohol poisoning. A helpful website is bloodalcoholcalculator.org. Put the website on your smartphone.

10. Stop drinking and leave the party at your pre-determined time OR when you or the people around you are getting drunk.
 This is probably one of the most important rules.
- Following this rule will help you reduce your risk of injury, sexual assault and alcohol poisoning.
- Be sure to stay with your buddy. Even better, stay with the entire group. Encourage friends who are drunk to leave with you. No girl should stay behind.
- Remember this: If the guy likes you, he will call you tomorrow when he is not drinking. Leave with your friends.

11. Never drink and drive.
- Call a taxi or take the school shuttle.
- Don't accept a ride from anyone else who's been drinking.

12. Help someone who is at risk.
- If someone is intoxicated, vomiting or passed out, they are at risk of injury, sexual assault, and alcohol poisoning. Do not leave them alone. This is an emergency. Call for help! Get the dorm resident assistant or call 911.

13. Recognize if you have developed a drinking problem.
- If you realize that you are consistently drinking beyond your safe limit, make a change for the better and reduce your alcohol consumption. If you can't seem to control yourself, get help from your college health service or call one of the alcohol hotlines listed later in this chapter. Take care of yourself before you end up getting hurt and/or addicted to alcohol.

Kailey

An older patient of mine came in for an annual exam and told me about something upsetting that had happened to one of her children. Her daughter, Kailey, was a freshman in college and had attended a party with her new friends. My patient explained that she had received a call in the middle of the night stating that Kailey was in the hospital, unconscious and not responsive. She had been taken to the ER by an ambulance, which had been called by an anonymous person who said, "a girl passed out at a party." The college student weighed 120 pounds, was intoxicated, and her blood alcohol level was 0.30. The ER contacted my patient because they found Kailey's driver's license in her purse and called the local police to reach her family. The mother was so upset with worry, confusion, and anger. She wanted to know how this could have happened to her daughter. She felt that Kailey would have known better than to drink so much, and she was suspicious that Kailey was coerced. The mom drove to the hospital in the middle of the night to be with her daughter while she regained consciousness. It took two days for this young woman to be stable enough to be released from the hospital. The college's administration found out about what had happened and required that Kailey attend alcohol counseling if she wanted to continue as a student at the university.

A Gynecologist's Perspective

Every year, this scenario with Kailey happens to hundreds of college students across the country. Tragically, many young people aren't as lucky as Kailey and die from alcohol poisoning. If you choose to drink alcohol as part of your social life in college, then know your limit and avoid binge drinking to protect yourself from alcohol poisoning and possible death. Don't let this happen to you!

Alcohol Poisoning

According to the National Institute of Alcohol Abuse and Alcoholism, thousands of college students are taken to the ER

each year for alcohol poisoning. According to Mayo Clinic, alcohol poisoning is a serious consequence of binge drinking. Drinking a large amount of alcohol in a short amount of time can lead to high blood alcohol levels and alcohol poisoning.

The symptoms of alcohol poisoning include:
- Slowed breathing
- Irregular breathing (10-second gaps between breaths)
- A drop in body temperature
- Pale skin
- Vomiting
- "Passing out"
- Seizures
- Choking on vomit, and breathing in vomit due to a decreased gag reflex, which can suffocate someone.

Very high blood alcohol levels can lead to coma and death.

If someone is vomiting, they need help. They should sit up to prevent choking. If they lie down, they need to turn their head to the side. To best help this person, you need to call for help!
If someone is passed out, they are in serious danger. You need to call for help! **Alcohol poisoning is a true emergency! Don't leave anyone alone who is exhibiting any of the symptoms of alcohol poisoning because they could die. Call 911.**

The Dangers of Challenging Guys to Drinking Games or Drinking Shots

Some women will occasionally use alcohol as a means of flirting. This is an unwise decision for many reasons and can result in harm.
1. Most guys can "out drink" most women due to several factors.
   - Women have less of the enzyme dehydrogenase compared to men. This enzyme is in the stomach lining and breaks down the alcohol. Therefore, a woman will have a higher blood alcohol concentration compared to a man after drinking the same alcoholic beverage.
   - Most men weigh more than women. Based on the Blood Alcohol Content info on page 133, the less you weigh,

the fewer drinks it will take you to become intoxicated and reach harmful levels. Women typically weigh less than guys and, therefore, will get drunk faster than men while consuming the same number of drinks.

- Women's bodies have a higher percentage of body fat than men. After drinking the same drink, the woman with a higher amount of body fat compared to the man will have a higher blood alcohol concentration.
- Female hormones can influence alcohol concentrations. Women may have a higher blood alcohol content right before their period, even when they drink what they usually drink.

2. Drinking games and shots involve binge drinking and increase the risk of intoxication and alcohol poisoning.
3. An intoxicated woman is in a vulnerable position, especially around intoxicated men, and at increased risk of sexual assault.

Risk of Sexual Assault

The following statistics are very important to understand:

- In a 2011 study of all freshman women whose biggest binge was four to six drinks in one night, 25% were victims of sexual assault in the first semester of college.
- Of the women who ever binged on 10 drinks in one night since starting college, 59% were sexually assaulted in the first semester of college.
- 50% of all sexual assaults involve alcohol.

Sexual assault on college campuses is a significant problem for women, and frequently involves alcohol and binge drinking. One of the most important points of this chapter is to avoid binge drinking! Refer to Chapter 17 for information on sexual assault.

How do You Know if You have a Problem with Your Drinking?

Try the tools recommended by the American Congress of OB/GYN to figure out if you are demonstrating "at-risk" drinking.

1. TACE

    T – Tolerance: How many drinks does it take to make you feel high?   (More than 2 drinks = 2 points)

    A – Annoyed: Have people annoyed you by criticizing your drinking?   (Yes = 1 point)

    C – Cut down: Have you ever felt you ought to cut down on your drinking?   (Yes = 1 point)

    E – Eye-opener: Have you ever had a drink first thing in the morning to steady your nerves or get rid of a hangover?   (Yes = 1 point)

A total score of 2 or more points indicates a positive score for at-risk drinking.

2. Alcohol Quantity and Drinking Frequency Questions

o   In an average week, how many drinks do you have that contain alcohol?

(Positive for at-risk drinking if more than seven drinks)

o   In the last three months, how many times have you had more than three drinks on any one occasion?

(Positive for at-risk drinking if more than one time)

What You Should Do if You are Demonstrating At-Risk Drinking

- Choose to reduce the amount and frequency of drinking alcohol.
- When you choose to drink, consume three or less drinks.
- Avoid daily drinking; even one drink per day is at-risk drinking.
- Talk to your school counselor.
- Go online or to the library for free alcohol education materials.
- Call a substance abuse hotline, listed on the next page.

Hotlines for Problem Drinking

National Alcohol Treatment Referral Hotline: 1-800-662-4357
(Federal Substance Abuse and Mental Health Services Admin.)
If you prefer to chat: www.addictioncareoptions.com
Families Anonymous (if your roommate is an alcoholic):
1-800-736-9805
Al-Anon for families of alcoholics: 1-800-344-2666

Final Thoughts

- Drinking alcohol is a situation you will face in college that requires thought and advanced planning to help you stay safe when away from home.
- Be wise, be careful, and make good decisions.
- You can say "No" to alcohol: 20 percent of college students are not active drinkers. Think of fun social activities that do not involve alcohol.
- Avoid binge drinking. It is associated with most of the serious problems women have in college.
- Stick to your limit. If you minimize your risk of getting drunk, you will be less at risk of injury, sexual assault, and alcohol poisoning.
- When you're at the party, focus on your friends, the conversation, and the music rather than the alcohol.
- Most universities have a system where you will not get into trouble if you call 911 for a friend in need, even if you are drinking alcohol underage. It is important to help anyone that is intoxicated or passed out because they are at risk of injury, sexual assault, alcohol poisoning, and death.
- If you are having problem with drinking too much alcohol and are demonstrating at-risk drinking, talk to someone about it and get help!

Service to Others

Wouldn't it be an amazing world if each woman could walk down the street alone at any hour of the day or night and be free of fear of assault, injury and rape? Wouldn't it be a better place to live if schools would educate children from a young age about the negative and unacceptable impact of violence toward others, and that it's not OK for parent, friend or stranger to harm anyone? As a nation and world, we could rise up and no longer tolerate domestic violence or sexual assault; and large-scale efforts could be made toward education, treatment, and prevention of all forms of violence against women. My dream is for future generations of women across the globe to reach their full potential by the empowerment of individual freedom afforded by safety.

Organizations Working Toward a Common Goal of Safety for Women

1. Global Fund for Women: www.globalfundforwomen.org
2. Rape Abuse and Incest National Network: www.rainn.org
3. Violence Against Women Research and Outreach at Michigan State University: www.msu.edu
4. It's On Us: www.itsonus.org
5. World Health Organization: www.who.int
6. The U.S. government: President Barack Obama advanced the protection of women by signing a reauthorization and expanded version of the *Violence Against Women Act* on March 7, 2013. The original act was signed into law by President Bill Clinton in 1994 and can be viewed at: http://www.whitehouse.gov/sites/default/files/docs/vawa_factsheet.pdf
In addition, President George W. Bush signed into law the *Campus Sexual Assault Victim's Bill of Rights* in July 1992. The information can be viewed at: http://clerycenter.org/federal-campus-sexual-assault-victims'-bill-rights.

Consider getting involved in your college's safety organization or supporting the cause of one of these valuable organizations to help end violence against women throughout the world.

Chapter 17
Sexual Assault Risk and Prevention

Carrie

Carrie left school after having trouble her freshman year. She was invited to a party that was hosted by her new senior boyfriend, Alex. She was excited to go because she would meet a lot of his friends. Although the kids attending the party would be mostly seniors, she felt comfortable and kind of "cool" because Alex was pretty well known. The majority of the people at the party were of legal age, and even though she was only 18, she decided to drink the keg beer and do shots with the guys. Carrie didn't really know her alcohol limit and drank three shots after having two beers, all within two hours of arriving at the party.

Although she was having fun and it wasn't that late, Carrie wanted to head home because she planned to study a lot the next day. Alex was in charge and couldn't leave the party, so he asked his roommate, Dave, if he would walk Carrie back to her dorm. She did not know Dave prior to that night, and he had a lot to drink at the party, but he seemed like a nice guy. Because Dave was her boyfriend's roommate, she agreed to him walking her home.

Once back at her dorm, Dave asked if he could see her room. He said he used to live in the dorm and wanted to see if it was the same room. Normally, she wouldn't invite a guy she didn't know into her room, but Carrie was drunk and wasn't making the best decisions. She didn't want to be rude, and since he was Alex's roommate, she thought it would be OK. Once inside the dorm room, he sexually assaulted her.

The next day, Dave told Alex that Carrie had "come on to him" and that "she was trash." Alex broke up with her. She felt ashamed, "dirty", and stupid. She blamed herself and never told her ex-boyfriend what had really happened. Carrie was depressed and distracted and found it more difficult to focus on her schoolwork.

Soon her grades were not what she had hoped, and she went home to try to figure things out. Carrie came into my office to have STD screening.

What happened to Carrie is an example of what can go wrong in college when there is alcohol involved. Drinking by students in college puts women at risk of sexual assault. The following statistics from the Journal of Studies on Alcohol and Drugs were covered in the chapter on alcohol, but I think they are worth repeating:

- In a study of all freshman women who ever binged by drinking four to six drinks in one night, 25 percent were victims of sexual assault in their first semester of college.
- Of the women who ever binged on 10 drinks since starting college, 59 percent were sexually assaulted in their first semester of college.

A Gynecologist's Perspective

I take care of women who have been sexually assaulted. Because of patients like Carrie, I have firsthand experience with how devastating sexual assault can be and how often it can happen to girls in college. This is one of the most important reasons I wrote this guidebook.

Sexual assault and dating violence are serious problems on college campuses. I want you to be safe and have a great four years in school. I don't want you to be scared to move away from home, meet guys, or go on dates. Rather, I want to you to understand the best possible steps you can take to protect yourself and stay safe in college.

Definition of Sexual Assault

According to the U.S. Department of Justice, sexual assault is "any type of sexual contact or behavior that occurs without the explicit consent of the recipient. Falling under the definition of sexual assault are sexual activities such as forced sexual intercourse, forcible sodomy, fondling, and attempted rape. Rape is a term used to indicate forced sexual assault and is either attempted or completed."

Acquaintance Rape

This refers to a sexual assault committed by someone known to the victim as opposed to an assault committed by a stranger.

Date Rape

This is a term frequently used to indicate that the assault was by a person known to the victim and occurred when the victim was intoxicated or drugged and unable to consent.

FBI's Comprehensive Definition of Rape

On Jan. 1, 2013, the U.S. Federal Bureau of Investigation made a newly revised, more comprehensive definition of rape. It recognized that "rape victims and perpetrators may be female or male; includes vaginal, oral and anal penetration by a criminal's genitals or an object; and recognizes that physical force is no longer a requirement of rape so that the definition includes victims who are vulnerable to attack due to being intoxicated or otherwise mentally or physically incapable of indicating a lack of consent."

Six Important Facts to Know about Sexual Assault

1. Sexual assault is a common problem for women.
   - 18% of the women in the United States have been raped.
   - 80% of assaulted women reported that the rape happened younger than 25 years old.
   - 19% of college women reported that they had experienced an attempted sexual assault or rape since going to college.
   - In 2006 alone, 300,000 college women were raped.
   - Women between 18 and 24 years of age have the highest risk for violence from their present boyfriend or partner. The estimates of dating violence among college students range from 10-50%.

2. Sexual assault often happens to a woman by someone she knows.
   - 75% of sexual assaults are committed by someone the victim knows.
   - 51% of female victims report the attacker was her present or prior boyfriend.

- 41% of female victims report the attacker was a friend or acquaintance.

3. <u>Alcohol is often involved.</u>
According to the Federal Bureau of Investigations and the NIH, alcohol is often involved in episodes of sexual assault.
- Drinking alcohol increases a woman's risk of being sexually assaulted. An intoxicated woman may be less able to resist an attack, and an assaulter may view her as an easy target.
- Many college rapists target victims who are drugged, drunk, passed out, or otherwise incapacitated.
- 50% of sexual assaults among college students occur after the attacker, the victim or both consume alcohol.
- Studies confirm that an attacker's misperception of the woman's degree of sexual interest in him is a major predictor of sexual assault. In other words, the man misreads the woman's intentions. Drinking alcohol increases the likelihood of that misperception, and thereby increases the chance of sexual assault. This is why it is important to leave the party when the guys around you are getting drunk. One of them may misinterpret your degree of sexual interest in him.
- College women who have been sexually assaulted report that getting drunk made them take risks that they would usually have avoided. Alcohol can lead to decision-making inconsistent with a woman's typical choices.
- Many women who have been assaulted mistakenly believed that the social setting of a party or bar protected them because other people were nearby.
- Alcohol use may increase a woman's risk of sexual assault, however, she is in no way responsible for the assault. The attacker is both morally and legally responsible for the action.

4. <u>Drinking games and doing shots increase risk to women.</u>
This topic was covered in the alcohol chapter, however, I think it is worth repeating: Drinking games can be a common activity on some college campuses and lead to higher alcohol consumption.

The norm for many college parties is to drink heavily, and many students accept getting drunk as part of "normal" college life. Some women like to challenge men to drinking games and drinking shots as a way of flirting. I would discourage you from this activity because most men can "out drink" women, and you would be putting yourself at risk of getting drunk, making poor decisions and being sexual assaulted. For additional detailed information about safe drinking habits, refer to Chapter 16. Instead of challenging guys to drinking games, think of a less risky way of flirting.

5. <u>Date rape drugs are used to assault women.</u>
   According to the U.S. Department of Health and Human Services, a "date rape drug is put into a woman's drink by an attacker to make it easier to sexually assault her. These drugs alter a woman's ability to think or act, often causing her to forget everything that happens after she consumes the drug."

a. Rohypnol (roh-HIP-nol)
   - A pill that dissolves in liquids
   - Newer forms can turn a drink blue or appear cloudy
   - AKA: Roofies, Lunch Money, Mind Erasers R-2, Whiteys, Rope
   - Takes effect in 30 minutes and lasts for several hours
   - Symptoms: drunk feeling, nausea, loss of muscle control, dizziness, problems seeing, sleepiness, blackouts
   - Illegal in the United States; used in Europe and Mexico as anesthesia for surgery

b. GHB (Gamma Hydroxybutyric Acid)
   - A clear odorless liquid, a white powder, or a pill
   - Can cause the drink to have a salty taste
   - AKA: Bedtime Scoop, Cherry Meth, G-Juice, Liquid Ecstasy, PM
   - Takes effect in 15 minutes and lasts three to four hours
   - Symptoms: feeling tired and relaxed; dizziness; feeling like being in a dream; problems seeing; nausea; memory lapse; blackouts
   - Legal in the United States for restricted purpose of medical treatment of narcolepsy (a sleep disorder)

c. Ketamine (Keet-uh-mean)
- A liquid or a white powder
- Aka: Black Hole, Bump, Cat Valium, Green, Kit Kat, Special K
- Takes effect very quickly
- Symptoms: loss of coordination; slurred speech; numbness; vomiting; you may be aware of what is happening, but you can't move; memory lapse; out of body experiences
- Legal in the United States for medical use; primarily used in veterinary clinics as anesthesia for animals

6. There is a "common scenario" of sexual assault.
According to the National Institutes of Health, sexual assault typically:
- Occurs on a "date" and involves one man and one woman
- Occurs in the man's or woman's residence (dorm, apartment or house)
- Alcohol is usually involved
- Preceded by consensual kissing
- Does not involve a weapon
- The woman believes that she has clearly emphasized her non-consent
- The man misinterprets the woman's sexual interest in him, often due to alcohol or drugs
- The man overpowers her, typically by twisting her arm and holding her down
- The woman tries to resist through reasoning and by physically struggling
- The woman usually does not contact the police after the assault

There are Physical and Psychological/Emotional Effects of Sexual Assault

Physical Effects of Sexual Assault
- Injury
- Pregnancy occurs in 5% of cases
- Sexually transmitted diseases

Psychological/Emotional Effects of Sexual Assault

- A victim often loses her sense of control over her life during the assault. This sense of control is difficult for many women to regain unless they get help and counseling.
- Anxiety disorders, including Post Traumatic Stress Disorder, can develop.
- Low self-esteem often results.
- Depression is common after an assault.
- Sexual assault can derail a college woman from her academic studies, making it difficult to focus and succeed, thereby impacting her future.
- Risk of alcohol abuse and drug use rises after the assault.
- Counseling is very important for healing and moving forward.

Five Rules to Reduce Your Chance of Sexual Assault

1. <u>Trust your Instincts.</u> If a situation makes you feel uneasy, leave and go to a place that feels safe. If someone makes you uncomfortable, move away from that person and go near people you know and trust.

2. <u>Practice Your Sentences to Get Out of a Threatening Situation or Avoid it All Together.</u>
   You need to have a few go-to responses ready to use if a difficult situation arises. Practice them ahead of time so that they are second nature to you.

   It's not the time to fumble through a protest when you and your new boyfriend are alone and things are progressing quicker than you would like. If he pressures you for more, have your sentences ready.

   If you are talking with a new guy friend and he seems to be misunderstanding your intentions and thinks you are sexually interested in him, you need to be clear that you are not interested and walk away. You don't have to be rude, but you should be firm. If rudeness becomes necessary for safety, then say what you need to say to get your point across clearly.

I have reviewed some of these suggested sentences in Chapter 1, however, I think they are worth repeating:

- "No!" (Use a loud voice with a confident tone. Look him in the eye. This tells him how you feel without ambiguity.) Then get up and walk to the door. No matter what is said to entice you to return, keep walking away.
- "No! I'm going to go and talk with my girlfriends/roommate."
- "No, I'm not ready for sex."
- "No, I don't want to have sex."
- "No, I just got my period, and it's always heavy. I need to go home!"
- "Eww, what is that bump? I'm not having sex with you because you have bumps down there."
- "I don't feel good. I think I'm going to throw up. I need to go home."
- "This party makes me uncomfortable. I'm leaving with my friends."

These sentences are just suggestions, and you should choose what makes you most comfortable to say. The important part is to practice them so they come easily to you. Be prepared in advance of college, and then review your sentences occasionally during your four years in college as you encounter different situations.

3. <u>Recognize that Alcohol Puts You at Risk.</u>
   - Know your limit, and keep track of how many drinks you have had (Refer to Chapter 16). Drink slowly, don't binge drink, and avoid getting drunk.
   - Be aware if the people around you are getting intoxicated. Agree with your friends to leave the party or bar when others appear to be drunk. Get out and go someplace safer.
   - Remember, if the guy actually likes you, he will call you tomorrow when he is not drinking.

4. <u>Avoid Exposure to "Date Rape" Drugs.</u>
   - Bring your own drink to the party. Get your own drink at the bar.
   - Don't accept drinks from people you don't know well or trust.

- If someone offers to buy you a drink, walk with him to order the drink, watch it being made or opened, and carry it back yourself.
- Keep track of your drink. Hold on to it, even when you go to the bathroom. If you realize that you left your drink unattended, then pour it out.
- Don't share drinks, and avoid group drinks like punch bowls. They may be spiked with a large amount of alcohol or contain date rape drugs.
- Avoid gelatin-shots offered at parties. They might contain hard alcohol with a high alcohol content or date rape drugs.
- Cover your drink so that no one can slip in a small pill, even while you are holding the drink. Hold a cup with your hand over the top. Hold a bottled drink with your thumb over the opening of the bottle.
- Pour out any drink that looks like it has an abnormal color, appears cloudy or has a strange taste. GHB can make a drink taste salty, and some forms of Rohypnol can make a drink appear blue or cloudy.
- If all of a sudden you feel drunk or really tired for no real reason, you may have been drugged. Get help! Find your friends, let them know how you're feeling, and ask them to leave with you as soon as possible. Have them take you to the hospital or school health service to be tested and treated. Be sure NOT to urinate (pee) before you go to the hospital because the doctor will test your urine for date rape drugs.

5. <u>Take a Self-Defense Class.</u>
   - I suggest that all women take a self-defense class before going to college. If you're already in college, sign up now.
   - Practice the moves you learn so they are second nature to you. Take a refresher class every year.
   - Self-defense class instructors suggest that you do not show other people, including your boyfriend, the self-defense moves you have learned.
   - See Chapter 18 for information about self-defense.

Be Safe in your Dorm

- Always lock your door when you leave your dorm room, even to use the community bathroom. Never go to sleep with the door unlocked. Be sure to talk to your roommate about locking the door so you are both in agreement.
- Lock your window, especially if someone could climb through it from outside.
- Talk to your dorm resident assistant if you find the main door to the dorm repetitively propped open. Don't give out the main door key to other people.
- Go with your roommate or a friend to the basement garbage bins, laundry room, and bike storage. These areas are often dimly lit and can be secluded.
- If there is an elevator in your dorm, take note of the emergency button's location on the command panel. If someone on the elevator makes you feel uncomfortable, get out at the next floor rather than riding to the floor of your room.

Be Safe Walking on Campus and in Town

- Don't walk around alone at night. Call the campus shuttle or a taxi if you need a ride. Program the numbers into your phone.
- Get directions in advance of going somewhere new, especially if you are traveling or walking alone. Use Google Maps in advance.
- Walk with confidence and look people in the eye. Attackers are looking for someone they can overpower. They are less likely to pick someone who appears confident and not easily intimidated.
- Be aware of your surroundings. Look and listen to what is happening around you. Don't walk through campus looking down at your phone. Don't walk with ear buds in both ears. You won't see or hear an attacker coming.

Be Safe Taking the School Shuttle, Bus or Taxi

- Have the campus shuttle and the local taxi phone numbers programmed into your cell phone. Add an app to your phone for the taxi service in your college town.
    - Uber, Lyft, Curb, and Easy Taxi have good reviews

- Read the campus map in advance so you know where you're going.
- Program the shuttle/bus schedule into your phone so you are not waiting too long at the bus stop. If you attend an urban college, many large cities have transportation apps for tracking the bus schedule.
- Look around and listen to what is going on around you while waiting at the stop. Don't be looking down at your phone; don't wear both ear buds and play music so loud that you can't hear someone approaching. Be aware of suspicious people.
- If a campus shuttle or bus stop is dark, go to the next stop. Don't get out at a poorly lit location.
- Call ahead to the campus escort service to meet you at your stop to walk you home if you are traveling alone late at night. Program the number for the campus escort service into your phone.

Be Safe at a Party
- If you choose to drink alcohol as part of your college social life, know your alcohol limit and stick to it.
- Go to parties with your friends, and leave the party with your friends. Prior to going out, agree with your girlfriends that no girl stays behind; instead, everyone leaves together. Have a buddy system so that each girl has someone looking out for her.
- If you are getting drunk, you need to leave the party. Don't leave alone. Have your friends take you home.
- Have money in your pocket (not just in your purse in case your purse is lost or stolen) so that you can pay for a taxi if you need to get out of a situation and need a safe ride home.
- Do not give out your personal information (address, dorm room, cell phone number, etc.) to an acquaintance or someone you just met. If someone asks for your number, enter his/her number in your phone instead of giving out yours.

Be Safe on a Date
- When you go out on a date, hang out in public places like coffee houses, sporting events, and in the college commons. Double date or go out in groups with your friends.
- Don't invite the guy to your dorm room.
- Don't stay overnight at the guy's dorm, apartment or house.

Be Safe Driving to and from Campus

- Keep jumper cables, phone charger, and roadside kit in your car.
- Pay for a service like AAA to jump or tow your car in case of emergency. One episode (a tow, tire change, battery jump) and the service will pay for itself.
- Always lock your doors.
- Have your keys in hand when walking to your car.
- Have a whistle and a flashlight on your key chain.
- Keep your gas tank full to avoid stopping to fill up late at night.

What to Do if You are a Victim of Sexual Assault

According to the Bureau of Justice Statistics, women often do not report a sexual assault to the police or authorities. After the assault, many women feel frightened, ashamed, embarrassed, and uncertain about why it happened. They often blame themselves. These feelings of shame, self-doubt, and fear can lead women to avoid reporting the attack to the police.

- In the U.S., 60% of sexual assaults are not reported to the police.
- Among college women, only 12% of rapes are reported to law enforcement.
- If a woman who was assaulted was drunk, drugged or passed out during the assault, she is less likely to report it. In fact, only 2% of the victims under these circumstances report the assault to law enforcement.

Get Help and Report the Assault

- Get help right away. Ask your roommate or a close friend to help you. Call the hotline listed on the next page if you don't have anyone with you or feel afraid to talk to someone you know. If you don't want to talk, use the online hotline to get help.
- Go immediately to a medical facility to get care: an emergency room will be well equipped to help you. Most laws use a 72-hour cutoff time to collect evidence of the sexual assault, but the sooner you go the better.
- DO NOT wash your hands, change your clothes, shower, bathe, wash out your mouth, clean your fingernails, rinse out your

vagina (douche), go to the bathroom (urinate or defecate), smoke, eat or drink.

- Call the police/911 from the hospital or school health services. Tell the police everything you know and recall. Remember, nothing you did, including drinking alcohol underage, justifies a sexual assault.
- Give the hospital a urine (pee) sample to be tested for date rape drugs. GHB is cleared from the urine in 12 hours; Rohypnol lasts for 72 hours. Remember not to urinate before going to the hospital or school health service so a urine sample can be collected to test.
- I would recommend that you call your mother or other trusted family member when you are ready for that conversation. That person will want to know so that she can help you and support you while you heal.
- Get counseling and treatment as soon as possible. Women often blame themselves, and feel embarrassed and ashamed. Counseling, support, treatment and time to heal will help you move forward in a positive way after a sexual assault.
- Realize that you can regain a sense of control over your life. Finding places to socialize that make you feel safe, and surrounding yourself with people you trust, are two important components to moving forward in your life.

Call a Hotline

Call the National Sexual Assault Hotline to talk to someone anonymously 24/7 about what happened to you and ways to cope and heal.

1-800-656-HOPE (4673)

Get Online Help

Professional help is also available through the National Sexual Assault Online Hotline. The counselors can connect you to the rape crisis center closest to your college.

www.ohl.rainn.org/online/

Final Thoughts

- If you have been sexually assaulted, it's not your fault.
- You are not alone; many college women have had the same experience.
- Sexual assault can happen to any woman of any race, religion, culture, and socioeconomic background.
- Sexual assault is a serious problem on college campuses. Take steps to minimize your risk.
- Before you go to college, think through not only how you can avoid threatening situations, but also how you can get out of bad situations that have already begun. Practice your go-to sentences so they're ready when needed.
- Since most sexual assaults involve alcohol, minimize your alcohol consumption and leave the party when you or the guys around you are getting drunk. Take steps to avoid getting drunk and exposed to date rape drugs. This will make you a less likely target of attack.
- Since the most common place for an assault to occur is in a place of residence, do not invite a guy to your dorm room or stay at a guy's dorm, apartment or house. You need to go home and take precautions to get there safely.
- Take a self-defense class before going to college. If you are in college, sign up for a self-defense course offered through your school or look online for a local opportunity. Take a refresher course every year.
- If you have been assaulted, get help! It is normal to feel afraid, but there are many kind and supportive people who can help you. Getting treatment and counseling are the best first steps toward healing and staying on track in college.
- Remember, the assault does not define you, so don't let it hold you back from your dreams. Yes, you lost control over your life during the attack. With time and healing, you can regain the control, move forward in life, and become all that you want to be.

Chapter 18
Three Steps for Self-Defense

I have two daughters, and I want to be sure that I arm them with the tools they need to be safe as they navigate out into the world without me. Last spring, when my older daughter was a freshman in high school and my younger daughter was in eighth grade, I signed up the three of us for a self-defense class called "Fight Like a Girl" being offered at my daughter's high school. I told my sister about my plan, and she decided to attend also. She said that she felt nervous in certain situations when she was out with her two little kids.

I found the "Fight Like a Girl" program to be amazing!
The course taught us the basic moves of self-defense and how to apply what we learned. Each of us practiced the different self-defense techniques several times with a padded police officer until we had the moves down pat. We were taught what to do in situations of being attacked from the front, back, side, and even if we were on the ground.

In the end, each of us had to "fight like a girl" and defend ourselves against an "attack" by a few padded-up policemen. While the other participants cheered in support, each participant fought off an attack by a policeman. One of my daughters plays competitive volleyball and is very strong. She was using all the moves she learned and fighting off the attacker, when all of a sudden, she used a volleyball hit, which landed on an area of the attacker that was not padded. He fell back coughing and winded. The surrounding women cheered as my daughter won the battle.

Since taking the class, not only do I feel more empowered and self-confident in my ability to defend myself, I also feel better that my daughters have the tools they need to defend themselves against problems they may encounter in high school, college, and beyond. My sister feels the same satisfaction knowing the self-defense moves she could use to defend herself and her children. I will take my daughters to a refresher course every year.

The Purpose of a Self-Defense Class

According to self-defense experts, the goal of a self-defense class is to "make defending yourself an instinct, not a reaction." Of course, you may encounter frightening situations sometimes, but the goal of a self-defense class is to not allow that fear to prevent you from protecting yourself. The police are not always around, so it's important that every college woman learns what to do in case of an attack and how to get away safely.

Sexual assault is not about an attacker wanting to have sex with a woman; it's about having power over her. So, one way to combat that is to not give anyone else the power. Practice walking with confidence; look people in the eye. Looking like you know where you are, where you are going, and that you know how to defend yourself is an important part of making you a less likely victim.

Three Steps for Self-Defense for College Women

Several of these tips are covered in the alcohol and the sexual assault chapters, but I think they are worth repeating.

Step 1. Get Prepared Before Going to College

- Practice yelling "No" loud enough for others to hear. This may feel intimidating to do, but it may help save your life.
- Attach a whistle and small flashlight to your keychain.
- Practice walking with confidence. Attackers don't want a confrontation; they want someone they can overpower. Even if you don't feel very confident, fake it. Walk with your shoulders back, head up, and look people in the eye.
- Practice "getting away from an attacker." The number one way an attacker gets a victim onto the ground is by grabbing her hair or ponytail as she turns to run away. While looking into a mirror, practice backing away quickly while facing an attacker, then turning at a safe distance to run away.
- Practice safely getting up off the ground. Leaning forward while you get up is dangerous because you are vulnerable to being punched or kicked in the face. While lying on your belly, move your legs back and away from your "attacker." Then push your upper body up and away as you quickly stand up.

Step 2. Take a Self-Defense Class

The ideal time to take a self-defense class is before you move out on your own to go to college. If you're already in college, no worries, it's never too late to sign up.

Listed below are a few self-defense classes and programs to try with descriptive information from their websites. There are probably several more options. Look online, check into resources at your library, and talk to your school counselor for local opportunities.

Fight Like a Girl Self-Defense Class: "Based on developing simple and effective responses to real life assaults applied in a controlled role-playing environment. Women who complete this program will have the tools, knowledge and muscle memory they need to gain the best chance of effectively defending themselves if they are assaulted."

The Rape Aggression Defense Systems: "A national program focused on realistic self-defense techniques. It is a comprehensive course for women that begins with awareness, prevention, risk reduction and avoidance, while progressing on to the basics of hands-on defense training."

Martial Arts Classes:
   a. Jiu-jitsu
   b. Karate
   c. Taekwondo

Kickboxing: Classes offer a focus on self-defense.

The key to any self-defense class is to fully participate and then to practice what you have learned. Select a class that has a "hands-on" part of the program, if possible, because it allows you to practice and realize that you are capable of defending yourself.

Step 3. Protect Yourself during College

- Be aware of your surroundings, both by looking and listening.
- Do not walk while looking down at your cell phone. Do not wear ear buds in both your ears. You will not see or hear an attacker approaching.
- Travel in groups, especially if you are walking at night.
- Make sure you have clear directions before heading for your destination, especially when going to unfamiliar areas. Pull up Google Maps onto your phone, use the iPhone app or print out directions in advance of leaving.
- Have money in your pocket and the number for a taxi service or campus shuttle programmed into your phone so you have a safe ride when needed.
- Agree with your friends in advance of the party that you will all leave together. If you are going with a large group, decide on a buddy system so that you know there is at least one person who will keep track of you, and vice versa.
- Do not binge drink!
- Take a self-defense refresher course every year. Look for classes near your college. Some schools offer self-defense courses as part of their curriculum.

Final Thoughts

I would encourage you to think seriously about how you will take care of yourself in college. Make a plan for safety. Taking steps to protect yourself will help you feel confident and stay safe away from home.

To be prepared, I recommend that you attend a self-defense class before you move away from home. If you are already in college, find out if your school offers a self-defense course or look online for local opportunities. Self-defense classes may sound intimidating, but they are very valuable in teaching you how to protect yourself, learning to get away safely, and feeling confident in your daily activities in college.

Chapter 19
The Abuse of Prescription Drugs by College Students

Lisa

Lisa came into my office during Christmas break of her freshman year. She was devastated that her friend had just died from a drug overdose on the weekend following final exams. Lisa had joined some clubs her first semester of college and was very happy and doing well in school. Because she became involved in the leadership aspect of one of her clubs, Lisa became friends with some of the older, more senior, girls, including Alice, her friend who had died.

Lisa explained that Alice was a very nice person and well respected by everyone. She was a hard worker, excellent student, and majoring in mechanical engineering. She had a nice boyfriend of five years, and Alice would talk about how they were going to get married. Alice had also been offered a job by an engineering company and was going to start work soon after graduation next semester. Lisa described Alice as someone who was "so together" and "had everything going for her." She felt that Alice's overdose just didn't make sense and completely surprised everyone who knew her.

On the night following final exams, Alice overdosed on Xanax and alcohol. Lisa learned that Alice was completely stressed out during the past semester, and started to take "just a few" of her roommate's prescription medication for anxiety. People knew that Alice was intense about studying and perceived her to be "just like all the other engineering students." No one knew that Alice was struggling so significantly with the stress of school or that she had started to take more and more of her roommate's prescription medication to try to relax. Unfortunately, one night Alice had taken too much Xanax and then had a few beers to celebrate the end of the semester. She stopped breathing and died. Her roommate found her in their apartment on the Friday night after final exams.

Most of the students returned to campus the following week for a vigil and memorial service for Alice. Many people stood up to say amazing things about Alice, especially her boyfriend and family. Everyone grieved the tragic loss of a woman with so much potential and promise for wonderful things ahead her in life.

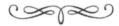

A Gynecologist's Perspective

Drugs kill people every day. If you take drugs in college, you could die, just like Alice. No one ever thinks it will happen to him or her, but nearly three people an hour die from a drug overdose.

Perhaps you've never thought about this, but as a doctor, it's unbelievably difficult to take care of a family who has lost a child to suicide or accidental death. Having helped parents heal from the tremendous grief after the death of a child, I know how loss can affect the people who are still living.

Families have a very difficult time handling the death of a child, and oftentimes cannot move forward. Arguments develop between the surviving family members who struggle to cope with the loss. Parents sometimes get divorced due to the grief from the death of their child. Kids who lose their brother or sister oftentimes become depressed and perform poorly in school. Many withdraw from their friends. Young adults, who lose their boyfriend or girlfriend to suicide, alcohol poisoning, or drug overdose, often blame themselves for not intervening and trying to make their partner change his or her behavior.

Realize that if you choose to take drugs in college, YOU not only harm yourself, but you also have a significant impact on the lives of the people who love you. If you die, many of the people in your life will truthfully fail in their own paths because they cannot cope with losing you. You have a responsibility to think about how your actions affect not only you, but also the lives of others.

I challenge you to choose to NOT take any drugs in college. If you are having a problem, then get help and talk about it. Call someone, anyone, to ask for help. No judgment. No criticism. Just call.

National Substance Abuse Hotline: 1-800-662-4357

National Suicide Prevention Lifeline 1-800-273-TALK (8255)

What You Need to Know about the Abuse of Prescription Drugs

Important Statistics

Alice's death is one example of the following sad, tragic, and factual statistics:

- The two leading reasons why college-aged students die are:
  - Accidents including injury, alcohol poisoning, and prescription drug overdose
  - Suicide
- Approximately 50% of college students report that they have been offered someone else's prescription medication at some time during college.
- According to the National Survey on Drug Use and Health in 2010, more than 11% of people ages 12-25 reported using a prescription drug when they didn't have an actual medical problem. They obtained the medication from a friend or drug dealer or they faked symptoms of a medical condition in front of a doctor in order to get a prescription.
- According to the Clinton Foundation, one person dies every 19 minutes from a drug overdose in the United States.
- The Centers for Disease Control reported that 38,329 people died from drug overdoses in the United States in 2010.

Reasons Why Students Take Other People's Prescriptions

- There is a common misperception among college students that a prescription medication is safer to take than an illegal drug.
- Many college students erroneously think it's OK to take other people's prescription drugs because a doctor has prescribed the medication, "so it must be safe to use." This thinking is a mistake.

- Some students feel that certain prescription drugs will help them perform better in school and therefore justify their decision to inappropriately take the medications.
  - Adderall and Vyvanse are taken by some students to try to stay awake to study for exams or pull an all-nighter. Some take these drugs just before a test to try to intensely focus.
  - Xanax and Valium are taken by some students to try to relax after an exam, reduce their stress from school or get high at a party. Oxycontin is taken to get high or relieve pain.
  - Sometimes, students will take Xanax, Oxycontin, or Valium to counteract the insomnia or intense focus caused by taking Adderall or Vyvanse. These students are on a drug roller coaster, which is very addictive and harmful.

What To Do if Someone Offers You a Medication or Asks for Yours

What Should You Do if Someone Offers You a Prescription Medication?

- If someone offers you his or her medication to help you stay awake or focused; to study, relax or reduce stress, pain or anxiety, just say "No" and walk away.
- Understand that once you start taking these drugs, you can become addicted and unable to control your need for more.
- Be aware that it is illegal to take a medication that has not been prescribed for you.
- If you think you have a problem with focus and attention, anxiety, pain or stress, then talk to your doctor about what may be happening with your body and ask what you can do about it in an appropriate and healthy way.

What Should You Do if Someone Asks You for Your Medication?

- If you are on a medication, then take it properly and keep it to yourself.
- If someone wants your medication, I'd suggest you say, "No, I need my medication. If you are having (illness), your doctor can help you." Then walk away.

- Do not give or sell your medication to other students. You don't know who will have an allergic reaction or harmful side effect to the drug or the dyes and preservatives in the tablet.
- You will be partially to blame if someone gets hurt from taking your medication. It is illegal, and considered drug trafficking, if you sell your medication to someone else.

Prescription Medications Often Abused in College

Adderall
(Amphetamine + Dextroamphetamine combined into one pill)
- This medication is a stimulant that acts in the brain to treat patients diagnosed with attention-deficit hyperactivity disorder (ADHD) who are overactive, cannot concentrate or are easily distracted.
- It helps people with ADHD to increase attention, stay focused longer, and decrease a feeling of restlessness.
- It is also a treatment for people with narcolepsy who suddenly fall asleep or have the uncontrollable desire to sleep.

The Abuse of Adderall
- Some students inappropriately take this medication to stay up all night to study or to increase their focus right before an exam.
- Abuse of Adderall is common among college students between 18 and 22 years old. Full-time college students are two times more likely to abuse Adderall compared to people of the same age who are not in college.
- One in five college students admit to taking Adderall without a diagnosis of ADHD.
- In one study, 60 percent of college students with the diagnosis of ADHD reported that they gave their medication, at some point in college, to another student who didn't have ADHD.

Vyvanse
(Lisdexamfetamine Dimesylate)
- This medication acts in the brain similarly to Adderall for patients with ADHD. It is a taken only once per day, which can be easier for students with ADHD to remember to take.

Risks and Side Effects of Adderall and Vyvanse

- Both of these medications have the same side effects of anxiety, aggression, heart palpitations, restlessness, bladder pain, difficulty urinating, depression, difficulty sleeping/insomnia, irritability, rapid mood swings, blood pressure changes, headaches, and loss of appetite.
- These medications can be addictive. Some people can get a feeling of anxiety if they don't keep taking the medication. Many become psychologically addicted and complain that they cannot function, get through their day or complete their schoolwork without the medication. Other students find that they need more and more of the medication to have the same effect.
- Both medications interact with other meds for depression/mood disorders. Mixing these meds with alcohol is very dangerous.
- **You can overdose on these meds and die due to an irregular heartbeat, heart attack or stroke.**

Oxycontin (Oxycodone)

- This medication is a prescription narcotic that works in the brain to reduce moderate or severe pain.
- It is to be used for a short period of time for patients who have had surgery or medical conditions that cause moderate to severe pain. It is not to be used for mild pain or "as needed."
- Long-term use can lead to addiction, both physical and emotional/psychological.
- Studies have shown that students who start taking narcotics at a young age often progress in their drug addiction to taking additional prescription and illegal drugs in the future.

The Abuse of Oxycontin

- Addictive painkillers, including Oxycontin, caused 75 percent of the deaths due to prescription drug overdoses in 2010.
- Overdoses of prescription pain medications kill more college students than heroin and cocaine combined.

Risks and Side Effects of Oxycontin

- Dizziness, lightheadedness, fainting, confusion, difficulty breathing, cold sweats, tightness in the chest, difficulty urinating, facial swelling, and trembling.

- Symptoms of an overdose include extreme fatigue and dizziness, slowed breathing, decreased heartbeat, seizures, and cold, clammy skin. **Often, people die from an Oxycontin overdose because they stop breathing.**

<u>Xanax</u> (Alprazolam)

- This medication works in the brain and nerves to treat patients with anxiety and panic attacks. It is in the category of drugs called Benzodiazepines, which are sedatives, anxiolytics, anticonvulsants, and muscle relaxants.
- Xanax helps people with anxiety and panic attacks to feel calm by increasing the effect of certain chemicals in their bodies.
- It is dangerous to take these types of medications if you drink alcohol frequently or have liver problems, alcohol addiction, myasthenia gravis, sleep apnea, glaucoma, breathing disorders like asthma or are pregnant.

<u>The Abuse of Xanax</u>

- Some college students use Xanax to relax or feel high.
- Some take it to come down from Adderall, Vyvanse or other illegal drugs like Ecstasy.

<u>Valium</u> (Diazepam)

- This medication acts in the brain similarly to Xanax. It is used to treat anxiety disorders, alcohol withdrawal symptoms, muscle spasms, and seizures.

<u>Risks and Side Effects of Xanax and Valium</u>

- Dizziness, increased saliva, change in sex drive, loss of sexual function, drowsiness, and memory lapse are possible side effects.
- Symptoms of an overdose include mental or mood changes, hallucinations, slurred speech, difficulty forming words, trouble walking, altered breathing, and loss of coordination.
- **Never mix alcohol with Xanax or Valium. This combination is extremely dangerous, intensifies the effects of the alcohol, and can cause you to die.**
- Talk to your doctor if want to discontinue the prescription. An abrupt stop can cause seizures and other medical complications.

Final Thoughts

- College can be stressful for many students. You are not alone. Talk to your doctor about healthy ways to manage your stress. See Chapter 20 for 10 suggestions to reduce stress.
- Taking other people's medications in order to manage your study habits, emotional status, and recreation is unhealthy, illegal, and possibly deadly.
- Do not take someone else's medications, even if it is offered to you or the person tries to convince you that the drug will help you perform better academically. Don't be misled by bad advice.
- Just because a doctor has prescribed a medication for your friend doesn't mean that it's safe for you to use or that it's safer than illegal drugs. If the drug were safe for everyone to take, it would be available without a prescription.
- Understand that prescription medications are intended for the person on the prescription bottle only. If someone without the medical condition takes the drug, there can be serious and harmful consequences.
- Many of these abused drugs are addictive and can make you feel like you need the drug. The addiction often worsens with continued use and can be harmful or deadly.
- If you are having a problem and need help, tell a friend, call your doctor, contact your dorm RA, or the student health service.
- Understand that your actions do affect the people who love you.
- If you have taken one of these medications and are having a side effect or allergic reaction, immediately call 911.

HOTLINES
National Substance Abuse Hotline: 1-800-662-4357
To chat online: www.addictioncareoptions.com
National Suicide Prevention Lifeline: 1-800-273-TALK (8255)

Resources for Additional Information
Centers for Disease Control and Prevention
National Center on Addiction and Substance Abuse
National Institute on Drug Abuse
The Clinton Foundation
The Jed Foundation

Be Happy

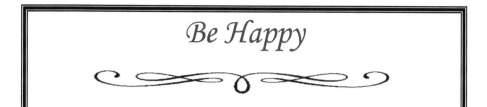

When I arrived at college my freshman year, I was like most kids—excited, nervous, and a little naïve. I had my new comforter, a mini-fridge, shower caddy, and loads of clothes. I felt reasonably prepared to study, but soon realized that I wasn't prepared for the freedom, the diversity of people, and all the distractions. I didn't have the same sense of control as I did at home. After awhile, I started to feel a little "down."

My roommate was a very nice and intelligent person, but she had a strong East Coast accent, and I had a difficult time understanding her. Music was often blasting at all hours of the night in my dorm, and a party could be found on campus any night of the week. There were so many guys walking around my dorm, which made it difficult to focus on studying. I stayed up too late in the first few months of college, which made completing my schoolwork more challenging.

With all these new experiences and distractions, I didn't really know what I was supposed to be doing. I felt insecure and uncertain about myself, and I wasn't as happy as I thought I would be. Was this what college was all about? Was I supposed to be at a party all the time in order to have a good time and make friends? How did studying fit in with all this fun? How was I supposed to stay on top of it all?

I needed some help figuring it all out, so I called my brother who was a sophomore at another university. He was an engineering major, getting good grades and having a lot of fun in school. He said something that stuck with me during my four years in college. He said, "Work hard and then go out and have fun. Do what YOU know is right, not what other people are trying to get you to do." He said the kids who were out every night were never going to make it academically. He was right—several of the girls I knew didn't come back to school second semester due to poor grades.

Years later, as a doctor, I find many of my patients have similar experiences in college. The patients who are always at a party and not committed to studying often don't reach their academic goals. The patients who study all the time and skip the social aspects of college are often stressed out. The girls who don't eat right or exercise often feel more depressed. Each of these women is out of balance and not reaching her full potential.

By listening to my patients, I find that the college-age women who work hard to stay on track for their goals, find balance in their lifestyles, and make decisions consistent with their personal values seem to be the happiest.

I'd encourage you to have a great time in college and enjoy all that it has to offer, but to try to avoid the distractions that could derail you from your path. Stay focused on your goals and find balance in your schoolwork and social life so that you can stay on top of it all and have the best college experience.

The following chapters will outline steps to help you find YOUR happiness in college.

Chapter 20
Ten Suggestions to Reduce Stress in College

College can put a lot of pressure on students, and it's important for each woman to make time to de-stress each day. Finding ways to let go of worry, unwind, and be in the moment is very healthy both emotionally and physically. The following suggestions can help you find ways to feel less stress and greater happiness in college:

1. <u>Choose Friends who You Enjoy, Not Stress You Out.</u> The people around you have an influence on how you feel about yourself and your college experience. Try to find friends who have a positive focus, even mood, similar values, and supportive nature. If someone is dismissive, judgmental, critical, or too demanding, consider moving on and finding a new friend.

2. <u>Schedule a "Personal Worry Session" as Needed.</u> Have you ever found yourself worried or stressed about something, replaying the details over and over in your head, only to find that you have made the issue into something bigger than it really is? You are not alone as this is a common problem for many of my patients.

   In order to break this cycle, schedule 15 minutes in your day to address what is bothering you and focus on that issue during that set time. Once that scheduled time is over, let go of that issue until the next scheduled "worry session" the following day. Learning to compartmentalize your stress into a set time and focusing on that one issue can help you resolve what is bothering you, be more productive with the rest of your day, and feel better overall.

3. <u>Keep a Journal on Your Night Stand.</u> Many students find themselves losing sleep over stressful aspects of college. Keep a notepad next to your bed at night, so if you wake up and feel stressed, you can write down what is bothering you. Tell yourself, "OK, now I've got it written down, and I won't forget to deal with it. I'm ready to go to sleep now, and I'll think about it

tomorrow." This strategy to stress management has helped my patients who have faced anxiety in school.

4. <u>Add Relaxing Activities to Your Day.</u> Listening to music, reading a book or writing in a journal can help you unwind during the day. Sit and rest in a place that makes you feel calm, such as outside in the grassy quad or by a sunny window in the college commons.

5. <u>Find Support Buddies.</u> Take a 15-minute walk with a good friend to vent and let out any daily issues while getting a little exercise. Having a good support system has been shown to help women reduce stress.

6. <u>Work Out.</u> Exercise can help you de-stress and keep fit at the same time. In Chapter 5, I have outlined a Step-by-Step Exercise Routine for you to try in your dorm room or at the college gym.

7. <u>Add Yoga to Your Schedule.</u> There is scientific literature documenting the benefits of yoga for stress reduction. See Chapter 21 for suggested yoga poses to incorporate into your daily college routine to unwind and feel great.

8. <u>Enjoy Yourself and Be Present in the Moment.</u> The old saying, "Take time to smell the roses" can be a helpful suggestion. There is literature on the benefits of "being in the moment" to help you reduce your stress. This technique, called mindfulness, encourages you to be aware of what is happening within and around you, and to acknowledge your thoughts and feelings. Consider taking a mindfulness class to help you reduce stress and find a sense of balance in college.

If your school does not offer a mindfulness class, you can enroll in a mindfulness-based stress reduction online self-guided video course offered through Sounds True and the Center for Mindfulness at the University of Massachusetts Medical School in Boston. To register for the eight-week MBSR online course, go to: www.soundstrue.com/store/mbsr-course

9. Use Breathing Techniques. Slow rhythmic breaths can help you relax. Steps for several techniques are outlined in Chapter 22.

10. Try Acupuncture. There is literature about the benefits of acupuncture to reduce stress as well as other medical conditions. Acupuncture can help you feel relaxed. If you want to try acupuncture, be sure to find a board-certified acupuncturist.

What Not to Do

Stress eating: Some women eat when they feel stressed out to make themselves feel better. Chocolate, candy, and foods high in refined sugar and simple carbohydrates are common choices made by women who want to eat to relieve their stress. Unfortunately, these choices are high in calories, can lead to obesity, and may actually make you feel depressed. Stress eating is a very bad habit to get into, so try one of the healthier habits listed above to help you relax and unwind.

When to Seek Help and Counseling

If you are feeling overwhelmed, your dorm RA, school counselor, and student health service are all available resources to help you through rough times. If you are feeling excessive stress and becoming anxious or depressed, you would benefit from counseling. Most colleges have on-campus counselors available to address stress and depression for college students. Call your doctor to see if you have a more serious condition that would benefit from medication or clinical counseling.

Final Thoughts

Over the next four years in college, you will find that different types of stress will affect you at different times during the year, and some of these strategies may work better than others to help you feel balanced and less stressed. Try them all, and see what works best for you. There is no right or wrong answer. The goal is to have a more peaceful and happy college experience.

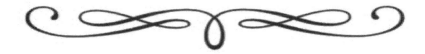

"Be kind to your mind.
Be kind to your body."

-Mary Dellanina
Yoga Instructor

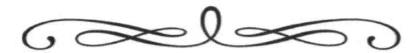

Chapter 21
Daily Yoga Poses for College Women

Yoga is a great addition to a healthy college routine because it helps build core strength, improves posture, increases energy, and reduces pain and overall stress. For college students who hover over their cell phones and computers all day, yoga is a wonderful way to stretch out and release body tension. Furthermore, it's a great way to disconnect for a while from all the text, email, Facebook, and Twitter stimulation coming at students throughout the day. In addition, yoga has been shown to improved focus, concentration and academic performance, and many colleges offer yoga classes as electives. Try these eight poses to help you feel great in college:

Combat the neck and back tension from hunching over your computer (and phone) all day:
- Mountain Pose (Tadasana)
- Camel Pose (Ustrasana)

Combat the imbalance in your body from carrying a heavy backpack on one shoulder while walking through campus daily:
- Downward Dog (Adho Mukha Svanasana)
- Tree Pose with Cactus Arms (Vriksasana)

Re-energize after a long day sitting in class:
- Warrior 2 Pose (Virabhadrasana II)
- Extended Side Angle (Utthita Parsvakonasana)

Disconnect from the world and de-stress:
- Standing Forward Fold (Uttanasana)
- Child's Pose (Balasana)

- Try the Step-by-Step "College Yoga Flow" outlined on the next page. This beginner level flow was designed to target the needs of college women, and can be done in the privacy of your dorm room or anywhere you feel comfortable.
- Purchase an inexpensive yoga mat online or at the local superstore.

- YouTube, yoga websites, and health magazines provide a variety of yoga poses to try.
- Two websites for a breakdown of beginner to advanced yoga poses are www.yogajournal.com (free) and www.gaia.com (fee). View instructional videos, read about different poses, and try the Sequence Builder to build your own yoga flow.

A "College Yoga Flow" with Step-by-Step Instructions

Caution:

If you have a recent hip, knee, neck or shoulder injury, do not practice yoga until your doctor has given you clearance. Always exercise within your own range of limits and abilities. If you experience any pain, dizziness, a poor sense of balance or have any medical concerns, stop doing yoga and talk with your doctor before further exercise.

"Yoga Flow"
o Mountain Pose
o Forward Fold
o Downward Facing Dog
o Forward Fold
o Mountain Pose
o Warrior 2 Pose
o Extended Side Angle
o Mountain Pose
o Tree Pose with Cactus Arms
o Mountain Pose
o Forward Fold
o Camel Pose (modified version)
o Child's Pose

1. Begin your practice in Mountain Pose, a fundamental resting position.
   Mountain Pose (Tadasana)
   - Stand up straight with your feet six inches apart, shoulders parallel to the ground, arms down by your sides, and palms facing forward. Slide your shoulder blades back and down.
   - Lift up your toes, fan them out, and lay them back down gently, feeling your feet form a solid base beneath you.

- Firm your thighs and feel your kneecaps rise. Picture energy rising up from your thighs, through your body, and out the top of your head toward the ceiling.
- Gently pull in your belly, and lengthen your neck upward to feel your head stretch toward the ceiling.
- Bend at the elbows and form your hands into a prayer position to rest the hands against the chest.
- Relax your face, body and mind. Be aware of your slow and gentle breathing.
- Feel your body in alignment. (What a contrast to hunching over your computer.)
- Stay in this pose for 30 seconds to 1 minute, taking five deep breaths.

2. Now reach your arms up overhead, and then swan dive into Standing Forward Fold.
   Standing Forward Fold (Uttanasana)
   - Step your feet together. If you are a beginner, keep your feet a few inches apart.
   - Bend forward from your hips and reach your hands toward the floor. Bend your knees to prevent pulling your hamstrings. Try to keep your back straight as you bend from your hips. Do not hunch over, round your back or roll your shoulders in.
   - Inhale, expand your torso, and feel your spine lengthen.
   - Exhale and gently stretch your legs and extend your torso downward. Do not hyperextend your knees.
   - Do your best and don't worry if your hands can't touch the floor or your knees are bent.
   - Hold this pose for 30 seconds to 1 minute, taking five deep breaths.

3. Keeping your hands on the mat, transition to Downward Facing Dog.
   Downward Facing Dog (Adho Mukha Svanasana)
   - Step your feet back about three feet from your hands or a distance that makes you feel balanced.
   - Spread your fingers wide and feel your hands firmly on the floor.
   - Push your hips toward the ceiling, head between your arms,

and try to straighten your legs. Don't worry if you have bent knees at first. Feel your back stretching long.

- Feel your biceps hug your ears, and keep your head aligned with your arms.
- Widen your shoulders and push your shoulder blades toward your hips.
- Try to push your heels to the floor if you can.
- Hold this pose for 30 seconds to 1 minute, taking five deep breaths.

4. Now, walk your feet toward your hands, back into the Forward Fold.

5. Roll up one vertebra at a time to return to the Mountain Pose.

6. Transition into Warrior 2 pose.
   Warrior 2 (Virabhadrisana II)
   - Stand in Mountain Pose. Exhale and step your feet apart, about 3- to 4-feet wide, with your toes facing the same side of the mat.
   - Raise your arms out to the sides, parallel with the floor, palms facing down. Reach your fingertips out away from your body, and feel your shoulder blades spread wide.
   - Turn your right foot out to point toward the end of the mat. Turn your left foot in slightly so you can stand with solid balance. Your heels should be lined up with each other.
   - Your right knee and right ankle should be in a line. Bend the right knee over the right ankle, aiming for the right baby toe. Try to make a 90-degree angle with your right leg, if possible, so your right thigh is parallel to the floor. Push your heels into the floor to help you balance. Keep your arms stretched wide.
   - If you feel strong and stable, turn your head to the right and look out over your right fingertips. (If you have neck problems or pain, do not turn your head; instead just look straight.)
   - Hold this pose for 30 seconds to 1 minute. Inhale and exhale slowly for five deep breaths.

7. Transition to Extended Side Angle Pose
   Extended Side Angle (Utthita Parsuvakonasuana)
   - From Warrior 2, place your right forearm on your right thigh.
   - Reach your left arm straight up over your head, palm facing in, to rest alongside your left ear. Shift your left shoulder back and your right shoulder forward. Try to keep your arm straight. Stretch all the way from your left ankle through your left fingertips.
   - Hold this pose for 30 seconds to 1 minute, taking 5 deep breaths. Inhale and return to Warrior 2 Pose. Then step your left foot forward to meet your right foot, and make your way back to Mountain Pose.
   - Repeat the steps for the opposite side, starting from Warrior 2 followed by Extended Side Angle, again returning to Mountain Pose.

8. Move into the Tree Pose with Cactus Arms
   Tree Pose with Cactus Arms (Vrksasana)
   - Stand in Mountain Pose. Shift your weight onto your left foot. Feel your hips center over the left foot.
   - Focus on a point 4-5 feet in front of you. Gently breathe.
   - Bend your right knee upward and grasp your right ankle.
   - Put your right foot onto the side of your left thigh with your toes pointing downward. Press your foot into your thigh. If you don't feel balanced or flexible enough, you can put your right foot onto the side of your left calf instead, or balance with your right toes on the floor instead.
   - Draw in your buttocks and "Root down," feeling the connection of your foot to the floor.
   - Bring your arms up, each into a 90-degree angle (cactus arms) alongside your head.
   - Maintain focus 4-5 feet in front of you to help keep your balance.
   - Hold this pose for 30 sec. to 1 minute, taking 5 deep breaths, and then repeat the steps while standing on the opposite leg.

9. Return to Mountain Pose and find breath.

10. Swan dive to Forward Fold, remembering to bend at the hips not in the back. Don't worry if your heels can't touch the floor.

11. Gently drop to your knees and make your way into Camel Pose.
   Camel Pose (Ustrasana)
   - Kneel on the floor with your knees as wide as your hips. Feel your shins push firmly on the ground.
   - Draw in your buttocks, belly, and thighs gently.
   - Put the palms of your hands on the top of your buttocks, fingers facing downward.
   - Press your shoulder blades down. Take slow breaths.
   - Bring your hips forward in line with your knees, open up your upper back, and move your chest forward. Draw your elbows toward each other and take slow breaths.
   - Keep your shoulders open. Feel your back and neck stretch.
   - Hold for 30 seconds to 1 minute, taking 5 deep breaths.

12. Find relaxation in Child's Pose to finish your practice.
   Child's Pose (Balasana)
   - Sit your bottom onto your heels. Spread your knees as wide as is comfortable for you.
   - Put your hands on the floor, palms facing down. Slide your arms forward away from your body so your torso comes to lie on your thighs. Rest your forehead on the mat in front of you. (If unable, rest your forehead on a rolled towel or block.)
   - Rest your elbows and forearms on the mat. Feel your palms and arms relax into the floor. Relax your neck.
   - Inhale and expand your back and ribs.
   - Exhale and let your body completely relax. Feel your body relax down into the mat.
   - Hold this pose for at least 1 minute, taking 10 deep breaths. Let your mind be quiet; notice how relaxed your body feels.
   - To return to standing, bring your hands back to beneath your shoulders and push yourself upward.

Final Thoughts

If, at first, you can't stretch into these poses quite right, don't worry because you'll master them with a little practice. Take your time and have fun. If you already practice yoga, this flow may be too basic for you, so take a look for more advanced poses on the websites listed on page 180. Adding yoga to your college routine will help you feel more relaxed and focused.

Chapter 22
Breathing Techniques to Decrease Stress & Feel Energized

A simple approach to reducing stress and re-energizing is to simply sit quietly and focus on your breathing. Literature has shown that breathing techniques can be helpful for stress management. Perhaps using breathing techniques seems silly or embarrassing to some women, but I'd encourage you to open your mind and try some of these techniques to help you re-energize, feel less stressed, and find greater happiness in college.

Three Breathing Techniques to Decrease Stress

Alternate Nostril Breath (Nadi Shodhan Pranayama)
This breathing technique brings awareness to breath, helps draw the mind to the present moment, and provides balance and a sense of calmness. The goal is to alternately press the nostrils while inhaling and exhaling slowly.

- Sit comfortably on the floor with your legs crossed. Place your left hand on your left knee, palm facing upward.
- Using your right hand with the fingertips pointed upward, place your index (pointer) finger and middle finger on the bridge of your nose.
- Gently place your thumb on your right nostril and ring finger on your left nostril.
- Press your thumb down on the right nostril and leave the index finger free from the left nostril. Slowly breathe in through the left nostril. Clear your mind of worry or stress, and focus on the sound and movement of your breath.
- Now, press your ring finger to close the left nostril, release the thumb from the right nostril, and slowly exhale through the right nostril. Pause and keep your fingers in the same positions.
- Now, slowly breathe in from the right nostril while keeping the left nostril closed.
- Close the right nostril, release the left nostril and exhale from the left nostril. This completes one round. Practice up to nine rounds.

Equal Ratio Breathing

This breathing technique can be done anywhere when you feel stressed to help you feel more balanced and calm. Try this in the classroom before taking an exam; prior to giving a presentation in front of a group; or during a study break while preparing for finals.

- This technique is most helpful when sitting in a comfortable position on a chair or on the floor. If needed, it can be done while standing or walking.
- Take slow deep breaths from your diaphragm, expanding your chest. Listen to your breath moving.
- Inhale slowly for six counts. Clear your mind.
- Exhale slowly for six counts. Relax your body.
- Do 10 repetitions.

Ratio Breathing with Longer Exhales

This technique is very helpful right before going to bed to help you relax and get a good night's rest. If you find you have insomnia, try this technique to help you get to sleep.

- Consciously inhale slowly from your diaphragm for four counts.
- Exhale for eight counts. Listen to your breath and relax.

Two Breathing Techniques to Energize and Refresh

Sometimes school may wear you down, so try the following breathing techniques for an energy boost to get yourself going again.

Equal Ratio Breathing with Retention

- Sit on the floor with your legs crossed.
- Inhale slowly from the diaphragm for six counts, and then exhale slowly for six counts.
- Repeat the same for the second round.
- On the third round, inhale for six counts and then hold your breath for two to four counts.
- Exhale slowly for six counts.
- Repeat for three more rounds.
- Warning: Avoid this technique if you are feeling tense because the retention breath can make you feel even more stressed.

Sitali Breathing

This breathing technique is a "pranayama" exercise, which many people find very refreshing. It is considered a cooling breath, and used when you want to cool down or feel rejuvenated.

- Sit on the floor cross-legged.
- Close your eyes.
- Form a slight "O" with your mouth.
- Stick out your tongue and curl up the edges (if you can't curl your tongue, no worries, just make an O with your lips and press your tongue behind your lower teeth).
- Inhale through your mouth and feel the cool air pass over your tongue.
- Exhale slowly through your nose.
- Breathe slowly and rhythmically for 3 minutes.

Final Thoughts

These five breathing techniques are easy to do and do not take much time. Incorporate a few of these breathing techniques into your healthy daily routine to help you unwind, manage stress, re-energize, and feel happier in college.

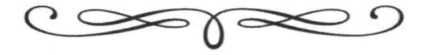

"It's a really exciting moment when you know something about the whole world that nobody else does."

-*Pardis Sabeti, M.D., Ph.D.*
Genetic Biologist
Sequenced the Ebola Virus

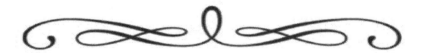

Chapter 23
Tips for Academic Success (and Happiness) In College

Whether your dream is to be a genetic biologist who helps improve the world's Ebola challenge, a world-renowned ballerina with the Joffre Ballet, or an author of a series of teen thrillers that are made into movies, you will need to put in a lot of work on the way to the top. College is your first step to getting there.

Reaching your potential is a very exciting process and completely worth the effort. However, achieving success in college is not easy and can often be very stressful. You'll need to learn some effective strategies to help you handle the workload while still enjoying college life.

Doing well in school will make you feel good about yourself and build further confidence, which often leads to a happier college experience. If you can adopt these five tips early in your college career, you'll be better equipped to stay on track for your academic goals, find balance and happiness in college, and get a great start to reaching your dreams.

Choose Your Friends Wisely
Making friends with similar values and goals for academic success is a helpful part of achieving your own balance and success. Surrounding yourself with people who are supportive and willing to put time and energy into their schoolwork will make it easier for you to do the same.

Learn to Handle Distractions
Since there are so many distractions in college, you will need to understand the power of "No" when faced with unhealthy choices and distractions. I found the following sentences helpful, but you should decide which ones make you comfortable. Then, practice saying "No" and mean it.
- "No, I can't go out tonight. I have to study, but would love to meet up with you this weekend."

- "No, I can't give you all my notes because I need them to study. Let's meet later to compare notes and study together."
- "No, I can't do your homework for you because I have so much of my own. Maybe you can ask the professor or TA for help."
- "No, I don't want to see the stolen test. You can be expelled for cheating."

Adopt an Effective Study Strategy

Learning to study is the most important part of academic success in college. The workload can be very heavy, and the tests are typically much harder and comprehensive than those you were used to in high school. Put in the time to really learn the material rather than memorizing for the test. Don't just get by, but instead put forth the effort to do your best work.

- Find a quiet place to study without distractions, preferably not in your dorm room. Do not study in bed. Sit at a desk that is relatively free of clutter, and your chair should have a comfortable seat with a firm back.
- Turn off your cell phone, as hard as that may be. It is a distraction, and you can always text people back once you have completed studying.
- Set an alarm clock to study for 50 minutes and then take a 10-minute break. Then reset the clock for another 50 minutes to study followed by another 10-minute study break. Stick to the schedule.
- To do well on a test in college, you will need more than one night to study. The best approach is to review each topic for 20 minutes each night on top of your homework. Then you will have studied all along, learned the material better, and increased your odds of a better performance on the exam.
- You will need to study at least a week for each topic to prepare for final exams. Cramming the night before will often be unsuccessful and can be very stressful.
- When you are in class, pay attention to the syllabus handed out by your professor because it is a guide to your teacher's expectations. Take notes in class, both from what is said and written on the board; your teacher will think both forms of information are important.
- Find a study partner to compare notes with and make sure

you have all the information you need. Form a study group to quiz each other and help you work through the more difficult material.

- Organize your room and backpack each night before bed so you can have a less stressful and less forgetful morning.
- Meet with your professor during his/her office hours. Although this may seem intimidating, your professor is there to help you succeed. Introduce yourself and show interest in the material. If you have questions, seek help rather than hoping that you'll figure it out. Be sure to have a clear question in mind beforehand. There are many people in your classes, so distinguish yourself by talking to your professor. This effort may open the door to future opportunities that can positively impact your career plans.

Schedule Time into Your Day to Put Away the Books

Taking time to let go of the work is important. If all you do is study, you will feel stressed out. The stress can take a toll on your body, and the imbalance in your life can make you feel unhappy. Make sure you get out and do something fun for two hours every day. You can workout, go for a walk, meet up with friends or join a club. Refer to Chapter 20 for some helpful suggestions to reduce stress in college.

Try Yoga as Part of Your Academic Plan

Studies indicate that students who engage in regular yoga have improved concentration, focus and academic performance. See Chapter 21 for a "College Yoga Flow" to add to your daily routine.

Final Thoughts

You have your whole life ahead of you, and doing well in college is an important part of forging ahead toward your future. Choose supportive friends with similar values because it's helpful to have someone by your side as you work hard toward your goals. Avoiding distractions is a challenge for every college student, but is completely worth the effort. Most importantly, find balance in your college lifestyle to reduce stress and enjoy yourself while working hard to reach your dreams.

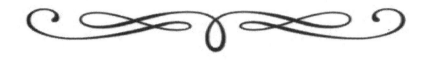

"A person who never made a mistake
never tried anything new."

-Albert Einstein

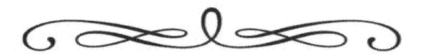

Chapter 24
How to Make Mistakes and Survive:
Three Suggestions to Help You Move Forward

You Will Not Be Perfect—That's OK

No one is perfect. Who doesn't make a mistake? I've made plenty of mistakes in my lifetime. No matter how hard you try, how much effort you put in, and how well prepared you think you are, things don't always turn out the way that you expect. That's OK, so don't be too hard on yourself. Recognize that you're only human, you just made a mistake, and the mistake does not define you.

Some of my patients get in the habit of thinking negative thoughts about themselves and feeling like they are a failure when things go wrong. Some may repeat a mistake even though it goes against the concept of the woman they want to be because they've convinced themselves that they can't do better. I've heard them say, "I'm never going to do it right anyway, so who cares?" I encourage all my young patients to break the habit of negative thinking and adopt a healthier positive attitude about their approach to life.

Three Suggestions to Help You Move Forward

1. Forgive Yourself
The first step to moving forward is to recognize that you did not intend to do something wrong, and that it's ok to make a mistake. Although you may feel bad about what happened, forgiving yourself enables you to let it go and try to do better next time.

2. Think About How You Could Have Handled it Differently
Rather than beating yourself up for making a mistake, turn it around by thinking about what happened and what you can do differently if the problem arises again.

- What about this situation led you to handle it in a way that was not consistent with your intentions?
- Why was the outcome different than what you wanted?

- Was there alcohol involved?
- Were you tired? Were you up late studying?
- Did you not have anything to eat that day?
- Does the person who you had the confrontation with consistently cause you stress? Does this person not have similar values as you?

If you recognize what went wrong, you can then figure out how you can handle it differently next time.

3. Keep a Notebook for Future Reference

Find a small notebook and take notes about the situation:
- What were the circumstances?
- What went wrong?

Write down how you'll take a different approach next time.
- "Before I have that difficult conversation, I will get plenty of rest and eat a big breakfast."
- "Before talking with my professor, I will read the material over and have a concise question in place before the meeting."
- "Before telling my parents that I don't have any money left in my school bank account, I will figure out where I spent the money so I can best explain my budget needs."
- "Before going to the next party, I will eat and drink enough food and water and stick to my safe alcohol limit so I don't become intoxicated and say things that I don't mean or make poor sexual choices."

Final Thoughts

College is a time of many changes, and you will make mistakes along the way. Don't worry—everyone makes mistakes. Forgive yourself, let it go, and make a plan for how you'll approach the problem better next time. A positive approach to handling mistakes will help you move forward, be your best, and feel confident and happy in college.

Chapter 25
Handling a Difficult Situation:
Learn to Not React

One night I was working late in my office. There were a lot of patients, and I found myself running behind schedule. I asked the front desk to call and notify the patients to come in a little later, but unfortunately they were not able to reach everyone in time. One patient who did not receive the advance call was an 80-year-old woman. She had already left home by the time the call was made, and she did not carry a cell phone.

Acknowledging that I was seeing her after the scheduled appointment time, I entered the exam room with a knock and an apology. What I received in return took me by surprise. The elderly woman stood up and angrily said, "You're late!" and then swung her cane and hit me in the side of the head. A small amount of blood welled on my forehead as I took a step back.

At this moment, I had a choice in how to handle the situation. I could start yelling, call the police and have her arrested for assault or I could take a deep breath and state firmly that her action of hitting me was not OK. Although I wanted to yell at the woman, I chose the second option. I told the elderly woman to meet me at the front desk, and I turned and walked away.

My receptionist was shocked and asked what me what happened when she saw the blood running down the side of my face. She told me to call the police. The patient came to the desk while continuing to yell at me that I should not make people wait. Recognizing that things could escalate if I didn't handle the situation well, I addressed the woman and stated, "Although it may be upsetting to some patients when a doctor runs behind the schedule, the intention is not to make them wait. Taking the best care of all the patients sometimes takes more time than expected. However, because you hit me, you are going to have to leave my office and find another doctor."

In college, things may be going along just fine and then unexpectedly a situation may arise that upsets you. There will be people who are unnerving. Others may annoy you or do something aimed at negatively impacting you. You need to learn to try to keep things positive and handle these interactions in a way that is in keeping with the woman you want to be.

Confrontation is not easy and very uncomfortable for most people. Learning at a young age to handle difficult situations in a calm way is a great asset to success and happiness in college and life.

The biggest challenge to managing a difficult interaction is learning how to NOT REACT. If presented with a circumstance that makes you uncomfortable or is confrontational, your initial response may be to react rather than to pause and think through what you want to say. Unfortunately, the reaction may not be a reflection of what you actually think nor in keeping with the way you want to present yourself. Learning to avoid reacting is a skill that will help you build and maintain healthy relationships in all aspects of your life.

How to NOT REACT in Difficult Situations

1. Get the Background Info in Advance if Possible
Gathering relevant details pertaining to the issue will enable you to understand not only how you feel about the topic, but to put yourself in someone else's shoes.
- Was your friend mad that you didn't invite her to the study group, and that's why she didn't tell you about the extra assignment given out when you missed class?
- Did the girl in your biology class think that you were flirting with her boyfriend at the party, and that's why she was rude to you in the cafeteria recently?
- Did you forget to call your parents for the first three weeks after getting to college, and that's why they're mad at you and won't send any money?

Trying to understand the details about why a particular situation is happening can help you decide how you want to best address the conversation prior to the actual confrontation.

2. Practice Beforehand with a Friend

The old saying "practice makes perfect" really says it all. Figure out what you want to do or say in advance, and then practice a few times.

- If you're nervous to talk to your professor about the fact that you were sick and weren't able to study for the test, rehearse your presentation with your friend before meeting with the professor.
- If you're embarrassed to talk to your boyfriend about the fight you had after drinking too much alcohol at a party, talk through your apology with your roommate.

What to do?
1. Anticipate what you may be questioned about during the confrontation.
2. Have the facts clearly in your mind.
3. Practice your answers so you can address the issues logically, in support of your position on the topic, and in a way that does not make the person you will be talking to feel defensive.

By being prepared, you will be less nervous, feel more organized, and avoid reacting if things become tense.

3. Have Your Sentences Ready

Take a deep breath before walking in. Have a few sentences memorized for an initial response. Some suggestions could be:

- "I didn't realize that. Thanks for telling me. I'll give some thought to what you've said and get back to you."
- "I can see you're upset. I'd like to hear what you have to say, but let's talk about this later after you've calmed down."
- "I understand what you are saying. Let's talk this through."

Although the person you are trying to talk to may be rude or antagonistic, try to be above it, stay calm, and stick to your practiced sentences. Keep it brief and try to keep the conversation on track to a positive outcome for both people.

4. If the Conversation Gets Heated, Stop Talking and Listen

Typically, people will argue their opinion with a goal of winning a disagreement regardless of the views of anyone else. This strategy may work well in a school debate, however, it's not the healthiest approach to a relationship.

When you're in a confrontation with someone else, try to ask questions, rather than repetitively stating your view. By listening to his or her answers, you'll have a better understanding of *why* the person feels the way she does and be able to put yourself into her shoes. Hearing what people say rather than repeating your own stance will give you a new perspective on the issue that you may not have considered.

It is not easy to listen while someone else is telling you something that you don't agree with. Although it may be difficult, I assure you it's worth the effort. This approach will allow you to find a middle ground for a solution that may be acceptable to both people. Furthermore, it will enable you to move forward in a positive, mutually respectful relationship.

5. Write Down What You've Learned for Future Reference

Keep your notebook updated about the difficult situations you've handled and the actions you took that brought about a positive outcome. A written log enables you to continue to evaluate and make changes as different scenarios arise.

Final Thoughts

Life is full of surprises, and you never know when a difficult situation may arise. The key to happy relationships in college is to learn to NOT REACT when a challenge arises. Think things through in advance, putting yourself in someone else's shoes. Listen openly and make decisions about how you will handle things in keeping with the woman you want to be. Using these five steps to handle difficult situations will help you be your best, maintain positive relationships, and approach challenges with confidence.

Chapter 26
Boost Your Self-Esteem in College

Moving out on your own to go to college is a very exciting time of your life! There are many new experiences ahead, and you will see the world in a whole new way. Although you may feel ready for all the fun ahead in college, you may also feel a little nervous or afraid. Sometimes the many changes that come with college may make you feel insecure and uncertain of yourself. That is normal. Realize that you are not alone, and everyone feels self-doubt occasionally.

You are going to change as you progress through college and become more experienced in the world. I'd encourage you to push aside your fears and welcome the change!

Every time you tackle a new challenge, you will have an opportunity to redefine how you feel about yourself and the direction you want to move in. The adjustments you make over time will continue to build on your best vision of yourself.

Recognize Your Success

Several of my young patients feel insecure, especially during their freshman year, and respond to self-doubt by asking their fellow students for feedback and direction. They look to others to tell them what to say, what to think, and what to do. In addition, they need others' reassurance that they did a good job. These women have trouble with their self-esteem and begin to rely on other people to build their confidence.

I encourage you to start to rely on yourself for your own positive encouragement and acknowledgement of your accomplishments. This enables you to build your self-esteem as you make your way through college. When going through an insecure time, you may tend to emphasize your failures, but I encourage you to focus more on what you have done well. Congratulate yourself on your successes. Be your biggest fan, acknowledging that you did a good job. Learning to recognize your own wonderful qualities and the positive actions you have taken along your path of life is an important part of making good decisions and becoming the best you can be. Here's how to begin:

- Look in the mirror and tell yourself, "I look good!" and walk out with confidence. You don't need anyone else to tell you.
- After you get a good grade on a test, recognize your effort. "I put in the hard work, learned a lot, and did a great job."
- When you've handled a difficult situation well, recognize what you did to bring about a positive result. "When I approached (name) with my concerns, I was calm and willing to listen. This made her less defensive, and we were able to work things out."

Although recognizing your own positive qualities may be uncomfortable for you at first, it will become more natural and easier to do with time and practice.

Think Positive Thoughts

If you're feeling down or uncertain of yourself and need a boost of self-confidence, read through the following list. After taking care of thousands of college-age women over the years, here is what I know to be true...about you:

You are special.
You are important.
You have something to say... and it's definitely worth hearing!

You will meet many people from all over the world and be able to embrace different cultures.
You can have an impact on other people's lives.
You can bring the value of your ideas to the world!

You are young and full of potential...
You can do anything you set your mind to!
You have your whole life ahead of you...
You are going to accomplish many amazing things!

So take a big breath, stand up straight and tall, and tell yourself, "Everything is going to be OK. I Can Do This!"

Think through an experience in which you needed to make an adjustment and were happy that it went well. Recognize the steps you took that brought you to a positive result. Review it in your mind so that it is easy to draw upon the next time the situation arises.

Jot down a few notes in your notebook so you can reference them in the future. Then, practice what you've learned:

- "I like how I handled the problem with my roommate this time, and I'm happy that everything turned out positively for both of us. I'm going to remember to approach that situation the same way next time."
- "My professor said my paper presented the facts in a more thought-provoking way. The hard work I put in to make the changes was worth it. I'll try a few new writing techniques next time and see if the paper is even better."

Final Thoughts

As you go through college, be open to the changes that make sense and move you in a positive direction toward your goals. Don't let fear hold you back from reaching your full potential. Instead, learn to recognize your wonderful qualities and successes and continue to build on those to move you forward on your path. There will be times when you feel insecure—that's OK. Every woman faces self-doubt occasionally, especially in college. Learning to build your own self-esteem will help you gain confidence as you navigate your way through the next four years. You are amazing, independent, and strong. So, chin up, shoulders back...Now, head out into the world and be all that you want to be!

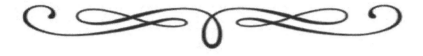

"Go confidently in the direction of
your dreams.
Live the life you've imagined."

-Henry David Thoreau
American Author

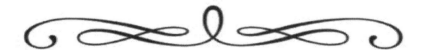

Chapter 27
Now Is Your Time!

College is the first big step toward your future. By reading this guidebook, you've now learned how to take care of yourself both physically and emotionally and are prepared to start the next four exciting years of your life!

As a graduate of college and medical school, as a mother, and most importantly, as a woman, I have three final thoughts of encouragement for you.

Find Your Passion

In college, I found it difficult to decide what I wanted to do with my life. In fact, I changed my mind several times about a career path - from an attorney, to a social worker, to an artist. Although I enjoyed many aspects of these different opportunities, none of them felt just right for me. I became a psychology major in my sophomore year because it seemed applicable to many different professions. Then, my father encouraged me to study for the MCAT and "see what happens." I gave it a lot of thought and decided it was worth a try.

Therefore, my senior year of college was devoted to reaching my goal. I studied very hard to get the best grades possible in my college courses and to prepare for the medical school entrance exam. I finally had a plan in place and a goal to work toward, which made me feel energized and motivated. These were my first steps down a path that really felt right to me. I was ready to jump in because I knew that I had finally found my passion.

Now it's your time in college, and I want you to discover your passion too. It may not be easy to find, and you may change your mind many times. That's OK. Just keep trying new things until you find your best fit.

Don't feel frustrated if other people around you seem to know exactly what they want to do after college. What's right for you is not the same as what's right for everyone else. Be strong, be yourself, and forge your own path.

You may find your passion when you least expect it in college, so be open to different opportunities. You will know you are moving in the right direction if you feel energized, find joy and satisfaction in what you are doing, and are motivated to be the best you can be.

Work Hard to Reach Your Goals

Once you have decided upon your goal, work as hard as you can to go get it. Don't go halfway there. Dive all the way in. Reach beyond what you think you are capable of. Even if you aren't certain of your exact plan, put in the hard work to move you toward your dreams. Whether it's writing a song, designing a building, planning an event, analyzing a financial plan or computing a chemical formula, find a way to do your best and advance the project beyond what it was before. Work your hardest and turn in your best work.

Surround yourself with supportive friends who are also trying hard to achieve their own goals. When you're feeling overwhelmed, commiserate with your friends, laugh off the stress, and encourage each other to keep trying. Our world will be a better place if every young woman succeeds.

Don't let hard work intimidate you. You are young, full of potential, and capable of becoming all that you want to be. College, like life, is not easy. Everything you really want may be difficult to get. Put your fears aside, and work diligently toward your goal. By working hard and putting in your best effort in college, you will learn the skills you need to meet the challenges of any opportunity you want in the future.

Bring Your Message to the World

College is an amazing place for you to find your own voice in our world. It will encourage you to think about your values, expand your views, and form your own opinions. College is a great environment to learn new things and evolve into an independent thinker.

Pay attention to current events on campus and around the world as you navigate your way through the next four years. Listen to the issues and really think about the pros and cons of each topic and some different ways to solve the issue.

Decide what you really believe in and what you think is important. Ask yourself what can be improved upon or changed, and then, most importantly, how you can make it happen. Believe in yourself, build your confidence, and develop your own ideas.

Each of us can have an impact in this world. We are not islands, but rather one of a bigger place. Whether it's an issue that impacts one person, your fellow students, dorm or campus, or an entire community, take your ideas and make them known. Pick a cause. Take some action. It doesn't have to be mind-blowing or record-breaking material. It just needs to be about who you are and what you stand for. Take one day, one confident step, at a time. Put your fear aside, and go out and tell the world your message!

A Final Word

I want you to make the most of your amazing four years in college. Be prepared, make decisions consistent with the best woman you can be, and take steps to be healthy and safe along your way.
You are young, full of potential, and can make a difference in this world, big or small. Get involved, find your voice, and bring the world your message!

I've given you the tools…
Now take them and go conquer the world!

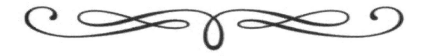

"Find Your Passion,
Work Diligently Toward Your Goal,
And Step Confidently Forward to
Tell the World Your Message."

-M. Susan Scanlon, M.D.
The Gyne's Guide

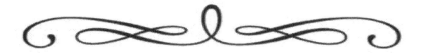

Addendum: Part 1
Helpful Apps, Wearables, and Websites

Apps to Keep Track of Your Period

- Clue - period tracker
- Period Tracker Lite
- Period Calendar/Tracker
  - My patients tell me that these three apps are helpful and easy to use.

Apps to Help Reduce Stress

- Breathe2Relax
  - This app helps you to use your breathing to reduce stress and feel calmer. It is easy to use and gives you a breathing schedule to follow. Try it before a test or presentation.
- Walking Meditations
  - This app helps you to reduce stress through meditation. The soothing voice tells you exactly what to do so you can redirect your thoughts and relax.
- Spotify
  - This app has many different choices of relaxing music to listen to. If you don't have a smart phone, go to their website www.spotify.com

Apps to Help You Get to Sleep

- Sleep Pillow Sounds: white noise
- Relax Melodies: Sleep Zen sounds & white noise
- SleepBot: sleep cycle tracker and smart alarm
  - Since you will need to keep your phone next to your bed for these apps, turn your settings to "Airplane Mode" or "Do Not Disturb" to stop the sounds of text messages from interrupting your sleep.

App to Help you to Remember to Drink Water

- Watermind Me
  - The key to this kind of app is to actually go and get a drink of water.

App to Calculate a Healthy Weight Range

- BMI Calculator for iPhone or Android
  This is one of the most commonly used apps among my
  patients of all ages.

App to Monitor Your Calories, Exercise, and Weight

- MyFitnessPal: www.myfitnesspal.com/apps
  - This is a great app to help you track your calories and
    exercise. It also has information about the nutrients in the
    food offered in different restaurants to inform you of what
    you will be consuming when you go out to eat. The nutrition
    database about many different foods is also quite helpful.

Apps for Monitoring Your Exercise

- MapMyWalk: www.mapmywalk.com
- MapMyRun: www.mapmyrun.com
- MapMyRide: www.mapmyride.com
  - These three apps are great to use for exercise monitoring.
    They track how far you traveled, how fast, and how long you
    worked out. The data is downloaded onto your computer so
    you can monitor your activity and compare workouts.
- Runkeeper: www.runkeeper.com
  - This app is a favorite of many of my patients. It tracks the
    paths taken, pace of exercise, and calories burned as they
    run, jog or walk. The distances and pace can then be
    compared over time.

Apps to Reference for Health Concerns

- First Aid by American Red Cross: www.redcross.org
- STD Treatment Guidelines:
  www.cdc.gov/std/tg2015/default.htm
- AIDSinfo: download this NIH app from iTunes

Websites to Help You with Healthy Eating

- SparkPeople.com: has a food and exercise tracker as well as
  motivational tips
- SuperTracker (from the USDA): helps you track your food
  intake; other tools are available to help with healthy eating
  www.choosemyplate.gov/supertracker-tools.html

Website to Help You with Yoga

- Yoga Journal: www.yogajournal.com
  - o If you are interested in adding yoga to your routine, take a look at this website. The videos will help you get into the poses properly and reduce your chance of getting hurt. If you have a problem with balance, it is better to go to a yoga class with a certified instructor instead. If you have an injury in your hips, back, neck or knees, always get the clearance from your doctor before doing yoga or exercise.

Website to Help You with Fitness

- Personal Trainer: fteamtraining.com
  - o For up-to-date information about the latest fitness trends, see this helpful website. It has a direct link to a personal trainer to ask questions about your fitness routine. Click on "contact us" to send your questions.

Wearable Devices to Help You Stay Healthy and Fit

- Fitbit: www.fitbit.com/compare
  - o This easy-to-use device is great to track your exercise. It counts and stores your activity, including steps taken, stairs climbed, calories burned, and number of active minutes.
  - o Log in to input the food you've eaten, and the Fitbit website will automatically calculate the calories, protein, carbs, and percentage of fats consumed. Compare your results to the food recommendations I have outlined for you in Chapter 2 to be sure that you're getting the right amount of nutrients.
- Mi-Pulse: http://www. mi-pulse.com/
  - o This new device is coming to market in 2016. It is a revolutionary sports bra that includes an integrated heart rate monitor for accurate calorie counting and zone training without the hassle of a heart rate strap. It's compatible with:
    - iPhone or Android-based smart phones
    - Leading sports watches
    - Various bike computers
    - Gym equipment that supports Polar

Reliable Websites

The Internet is full of information, but not all websites are reliable. Many of my patients come into the office with fear and worry after reviewing inaccurate information from unreliable websites. For up-to-date and accurate health information, I refer my patients to the websites below:

- American Congress of OB GYN: www.acog.org
- Mayo Clinic: www.mayoclinic.org
- Cleveland Clinic: my.clevelandclinic.org
- American Heart Association: http://www.heart.org/HEARTORG/
- USDA ChooseMyPlate.Gov: www.choosemyplate.gov
- National Institute on Mental Health: http://www.nimh.nih.gov/index.shtml
- Centers for Disease Control: www.cdc.gov
- National Institutes of Health: www.nih.gov
- Academy of Nutrition and Dietetics: www.eatright.org

Addendum: Part 2
Checklists and Questions to Answer

Now that you're about to head off to college, you'll want to be sure you have everything you need to be prepared. Some college checklists are based on comforters and backpacks; this list is based on keeping you healthy, safe, and happy when you move away from home.

Be prepared. Check off each item on this list and answer each question honestly—feel free to write your answers on a separate piece of paper. Be sure that you aren't one of the women who need to come into my office after Thanksgiving.

Numbers to Program into Your Cell Phone:
☐ Your family at home
☐ Any family or family friends living near your college
☐ Your family doctor at home
☐ Your gynecologist
☐ The school health center
☐ Your dorm resident assistant
☐ Your college counselor
☐ Your roommate
☐ School shuttle/bus service
☐ Local taxi service
☐ In case of emergency contact
☐ Bank
☐ Credit card company

Apps to Download:
☐ A period tracker
☐ Stress reduction
☐ Sleep app
☐ Calorie counter
☐ Water reminder
☐ Exercise tracker/fitness app
☐ First aid
☐ Study timer
☐ Google Maps, iPhone Maps or other navigation app
☐ Taxi service & public transportation

Info to Program into Your Phone:

- ☐ Academic schedule
- ☐ Cafeteria menu
- ☐ Exercise plan: 2 ½ hours per week
- ☐ The One-Month Exercise Schedule on page 58
- ☐ Campus bus/shuttle schedule & campus escort service
- ☐ Blood Alcohol Calculator website on page 133
- ☐ A general health file to store important info: including immunizations; health history; medication name(s), dose and dosage schedule(s); important family medical history
- ☐ Relevant hotlines

For Your Well-Being:

- ☐ Name three boundaries that are important to you to discuss with your roommate.
- ☐ Have you thought about your "best self" and identified your values?
- ☐ How much sleep do you need each night?
- ☐ List two things you can do to combat insomnia.
- ☐ How much water do you need to drink daily?
- ☐ Where do you plan to study?
- ☐ Name three things you can do to reduce stress.
- ☐ Try the Step-by-Step College Yoga Flow (Chapter 21).
- ☐ Practice a few breathing techniques (Chapter 22).
- ☐ Answer the questions about sexuality on page 92.
- ☐ Review sentences to handle a difficult situation (Chapter 25).
- ☐ Take a picture of the list of positive thoughts on page 200.
- ☐ Buy a notebook to jot down ideas to help you move forward after a mistake, to remember how you handled a difficult situation well, to reduce stress, to tackle anxiety and insomnia, and to build your own self-esteem.

For Your Medical Health:

- ☐ Schedule a pre-college check-up with your doctor or gynecologist.
- ☐ Get vaccinated for HPV, if recommended by your doctor.
- ☐ Get vaccinated for hepatitis B, if you're not immune.
- ☐ If you will be sexually active, get a prescription for contraception.
- ☐ If you will be sexually active, purchase condoms.
- ☐ Get a dental check-up and cleaning.
- ☐ Take a picture of the Bladder Irritants List on page 70.
- ☐ Review the products that can mimic a yeast infection on page 66.

For Your Safety:
☐ Write three escape sentences to use when needed (Chapter 1)
☐ Practice saying your three sentences loudly in a confident voice.
☐ Practice yelling "No!"
☐ Put a whistle and flashlight on your key chain.
☐ Take a self-defense class; schedule a follow-up class a year later.
☐ Put jumper cables, a phone charger, and roadside kit in your car. Consider joining a roadside assistance service.
☐ What three things can help you prevent STDs?
☐ Review the Blood Alcohol Content information on page 133. What is your alcohol limit? What is binge drinking?
☐ Know the three Steps for Safe Drinking (Chapter 16).

For Your Nutritional Health:
☐ Buy a healthy multivitamin, preferably from a whole foods store.
☐ Identify your healthy weight range with the Body Mass Index chart (page 38) or reference an online BMI calculator.
☐ Know the amount of calories, protein, grains, fruits, veggies, dairy and fat you need based on your age and level of activity (Chapter 2). Take a picture of the Food Guidelines on pages 22-23.
☐ Practice looking at food labels for calories, protein, sugar, fat and sodium. Know the recommended limits of each (pages 22-23).
☐ Take a picture of the Healthy Foods List (page 31) and the Food/Drinks to Minimize and Avoid Lists (page 41).
☐ Review the food high in iron and Vit. C to avoid anemia (page 79).
☐ Take a picture of the Strategy to Avoid Gaining Weight (page 39).
☐ Select the food items that fit your needs from the Dorm Room Basics List (page 31).
☐ Buy or rent a mini-fridge with a freezer.
☐ Consider buying a Magic Bullet or other small blender.
☐ Buy small storage containers and freezer bags.

For Exercise:
☐ Pick a few enjoyable types of exercise to do for 2 ½ hours each week (Chapter 4); put your exercise plan on your schedule.
☐ Try the Step-by-Step Exercise Routines for your dorm and college gym before going to college (Chapter 5).
☐ Try the One-Month Workout Plan before college. Mix it up to keep it fun (Chapter 5).
☐ Consider buying a Fitbit or mi-pulse sports bra to monitor exercise.

Addendum: Part 3
HOTLINES

CRISES AND SUICIDE
National Hopeline Network: 1-800-SUICIDE (784-2433)
National Suicide Prevention Lifeline: 1-800-273-TALK (8255)
National Youth Crisis Hotline: 1-800-442-HOPE (4673)

ALCOHOL
National Alcohol Treatment Referral Hotline 1-800-662-4357
Al-Anon for Families of Alcoholics: 1-800-344-2666
If you prefer to chat online: National Alcoholism and Substance
Abuse Information Center. www.addictioncareoptions.com

DRUGS
Cocaine Anonymous: 1-800-347-8998
National Drug Abuse Hotline: 1-800-662-4357
If you prefer to chat online: National Alcoholism and Substance
Abuse Information Center. www.addictioncareoptions.com

DOMESTIC VIOLENCE (boyfriend, spouse, partner)
National Domestic Violence Hotline: 1-800-799-7233
TTY for hearing impaired: 1-800-787-3244 (video relay available)
Chat feature online: www.thehotline.org

HEALTH TOPICS
CDC Health Topics Hotline (immunizations, health issues, etc.):
1-800-CDC-INFO (800-232-4636)
The Centers for Disease Control's help center will not answer any
specific clinical questions, but will answer general questions about
health topics.

RAPE AND SEXUAL ASSAULT
National Sexual Assault Hotline: 1-800-656-HOPE (4673) or
1-800-799-7233. You will be connected automatically to a local help
center. The counselors are available to talk with you 24/7.
(This organization was previously called RAINN.)

PREGNANCY
Your OB-GYN is the best resource for pregnancy. Give your doctor a call!

SEXUALLY TRANSMITTED DISEASE INFORMATION:
CDC Info: 1-800-232-4636
TTY: 1-888-232-6348
Operators will answer general questions, not specific clinical information.

AIDS
CDC AIDS Information: 1-800-232-4636
Health Resources and Services Administration: Go to www.hab.hrsa.gov/gethelp/statehotlines.html for a hotline number for the state you're living in.

EATING DISORDERS
National Eating Disorders Association Hotline: 1-800-931-2237
To chat online: www.nationaleatingdisorders.org/find-help-support

POISON CONTROL
American Association of Poison Control Centers: 1-800-222-1222

Acknowledgements

There are many people to whom I owe a great deal of gratitude. This guidebook took two years to complete, none of which I could have done without the kindness, support, and insight of the following wonderful people:

My family has encouraged me to bring my message to the world. They always remind me that I can do anything that I put my mind to and then stand behind me so that I can actually make it happen. Katy and Meghan, who I love so dearly, are my future college women and for whom this book is so carefully written. And my son, Patrick, who has forged ahead in college and makes me so proud.

My editors are fantastic! Suzanne Reeves, from Spunky Texas Publications, has helped me bring this book to life—I couldn't have done it without her! She believes in my purpose and has helped me stay on track for keeping my message throughout the book. Kevin Beese from BZ & Associates edited the book for the update in 2016. His work is detailed, thorough and completely indispensable!

My three college editors are truly inspirational women and future leaders in our world.
Emily Scanlon, my niece and a senior at St Mary's College, truly exemplifies a woman at her best. She met with me in the very beginning to pick the topics for this book. She will be a fantastic speech pathologist and mother. I can't wait to see her career unfold!
Aleksandra Ivanisevic, a freshman at Iowa State University, is an insightful young woman with an outstanding future in whatever career path she chooses.
Allison Hartnett, a recent graduate of Notre Dame, and the glue of the book, brought everything together through her formatting skills and thought-provoking suggestions. I truthfully could not have completed this book without her. She is an outstanding young woman who will definitely make a difference in this world.
Additionally, Hannah Winter, a scholarship athlete at University of Illinois, modeled for the exercise pictures. Beyond her impressive physical fitness, Hannah's intelligence and kind nature will continue to lead her forward toward an amazing future.

Three professional women edited my exercise, yoga, and nutritional chapters. These intelligent, hard-working women are fully committed to helping people achieve optimal wellness, and share in my vision for better health information for women. I am so appreciative of all their time, edits and suggestions. I couldn't have completed this guidebook without them!
Amy Winter, NASM Personal Trainer, ACE Personal Trainer & Group Exercise Instructor, MS Aquatics & AEA Aquatic Exercise Instructor.
Mary Dellanina, Yoga Instructor, E-RYT 200, Pilates Mat and Reformer Certified, AFAA Certified.
Susan Rizzo, RD, LDN, CDE, Licensed Dietitian Nutritionist, with Certificate in Adult, Child & Adolescent Weight Management.

My sisters, Kate, Beth, and Margaret, and my sister-in-law, Julie, have been a wonderful source of insight and encouragement. Beth was one of the first women I talked to about writing this book, and she encouraged me to forge ahead. She also made many suggestions as I tried to keep my message clear throughout the book. Each of these women has a daughter or two who will be going off to college and therefore had helpful insights into the various topics in this guidebook. My four sisters are kind, fun, and intelligent, and each exemplifies a woman at her best. Their support and friendship remind me that no matter what I do, they like me just as I am.

My two nieces, Abbie and Marianne, were also a big help to me. Abbie's careful consideration of the cover design, and Marianne's helpful editorial suggestions, helped me bring The Gyne's Guide to life.

My brother-in-law, Dr. Peter Schraeder, a professor and author, was an important part of confirming the accuracy of this guidebook.

And last, but not least, my mother, Marianne Scanlon—the eternal cheerleader. Her sense of humor has helped me keep going when I felt that I had taken on too much. Her optimistic view and supportive encouragement throughout my life has been my foundation to be the best woman I can be.

Thank you!
xoxo

References

"Abnormal Menstruation." Cleveland Clinic. April 2015.
my.clevelandclinic.org/health/healthy_living/hic_Coping_with_Fam
ilies_and_Careers/hic_Normal_Menstruation/hic-abnormal-
menstruation

"Abnormal Uterine Bleeding." *American College of Obstetrics and Gynecology
FAQ* 095th ser. (2012). www.acog.org/Patients/FAQs/Abnormal-
Uterine-Bleeding

"Addressing Health Risks of Noncoital Sexual Activity." *American College of
Obstetrics and Gynecology Committee Opinion* Number 582 (2013).
www.acog.org/Resources-And-Publications/Committee-
Opinions/Committee-on-Adolescent-Health-Care/Addressing-
Health-Risks-of-Noncoital-Sexual-Activity

"Adolescents and Long-Acting Reversible Contraception." *American College
of Obstetrics and Gynecology Committee Opinion* Number 539
(2012). Print.

"Adult Health." Self-esteem Check: Too Low, Too High or Just Right? Mayo
Clinic, 2015. www.mayoclinic.org/healthy-lifestyle/adult-
health/in-depth/self-esteem/art-20047976

"Adult Health." *Sleep Tips*. Mayo Clinic, June 2014.
www.mayoclinic.org/healthy-lifestyle/adult-health/in-
depth/sleep/art-20048379

"AHA Fat Translator." *American Heart Association.*
www.heart.org/myfats/fats_results.html?age=22&gender=2&weig
ht=125&heightfeet=5&heightinch=7&activity=2&

"AHA Recommendations for Exercise in Adults." *American Heart
Association*. American Heart Association, 2015.
www.heart.org/HEARTORG/GettingHealthy/PhysicalActivity/Fitn
essBasics/American-Heart-Association-Recommendations-for-

Physical-Activity-in-Adults_UCM_307976_Article.jsp

pubs.niaaa.nih.gov/publications/arh25-1/43-51.htm

"Alcohol Consumption Increases Women's Vulnerability to Sexual
Victimization." *National Institute of Health.* 2009
www.ncbi.nlm.nih.gov/pmc/articles/PMC2784921/

"Alcohol's Effects." Campus Alcohol Abuse Prevention Center. *Virginia Tech.*
2015. www.alcohol.vt.edu/Students/Alcohol_effects/index.

"Alcohol Overdose: The Dangers of Drinking Too Much." *National Institute
of Alcohol Abuse and Alcoholism.* April 2015.
pubs.niaaa.nih.gov/publications/AlcoholOverdoseFactsheet/Overd
osefact.htm

"Alcohol Use Increases the Risk of Sexual Assault." *National Institute of
Justice.* Oct. 2014. www.nij.gov/topics/crime/rape-sexual-
violence/campus/pages/alcohol.aspx

Antonia, Abbey. "Alcohol and Sexual Assault." *Alcohol and Sexual Assault.*
National Institutes of Health. Oct. 2014.
pubs.niaaa.nih.gov/publications/arh25-1/43-51.htm

"At-Risk Drinking and Alcohol Dependence: Obstetric and Gynecologic
Implications." *American College of Obstetrics and Gynecology
Committee Opinion* Number 496 (2013). www.acog.org/Resources-
And-Publications/Committee-Opinions/Committee-on-Health-
Care-for-Underserved-Women/At-Risk-Drinking-and-Alcohol-
Dependence-Obstetric-and-Gynecologic-Implications

"Avoiding Dangerous Situations | RAINN | Rape, Abuse and Incest National
Network." *Avoiding Dangerous Situations | RAINN | Rape, Abuse and
Incest National Network.* 14 Oct. 2014. https://rainn.org/get-
information/sexual-assault-prevention/avoiding-dangerous-
situations

"Beginners How to: Yoga." *YogaJournal.com.* 2015. www.yogajournal.com

"Binge Drinking by College Freshman Women Tied to Sexual Assault Risk, According to New Research." - *University of Buffalo.* www.buffalo.edu/news/releases/2011/12/13063.ht

Blood Alcohol Calculator Website. bloodalcoholcalculator.org/#LinkURL

"Breathe Easy: Relax with Pranayama." Yoga Journal. 2012 www.yogajournal.com/article/practice-section/healing-breath/

"Campus Sexual Assault Bill of Rights." clerycenter.org/federal-campus-sexual-assault-victims'-bill-rights

"CDC Fact Sheets on STDs." *Centers for Disease Control and Prevention.* Centers for Disease Control and Prevention, 09 Mar. 2015. www.cdc.gov/std/

"Certain Self-Defense Actions can Decrease Risk." *National Institute of Justice.* October 2008. www.nij.gov/topics/crime/rape-sexual-violence/campus/pages/decrease-risk.aspx

"Condom Fact Sheet." *Center for Disease Control and Prevention.* CDC. March 2013. www.cdc.gov/condomeffectiveness/brief.html

"Contraception." *Centers for Disease Control and Prevention.* Centers for Disease Control and Prevention, 24 Feb. 2015. www.cdc.gov/reproductivehealth/unintendedpregnancy/contraception.htm

"Date Rape Drug Fact Sheet." *Office on Women's Health.* U.S. Dept. of Health and Human Services. July 2012. www.womenshealth.gov/publications/our-publications/fact-sheet/date-rape-drugs.html

"Depression." *NIMH RSS.* National Institute of Mental Health. Web. 14 Apr. 2015. www.nimh.nih.gov/health/topics/depression/index.shtml

"Dextroamphetamine and Amphetamine." Mayo Clinic. 2015
www.mayoclinic.org/drugs-upplements/extroamphetamine-and-
amphetamine-oral-rout/description/drg-20071758

"Dietary Guidelines for Americans 2015-2020" U.S. Department of Health
and Human Services and U.S. Department of Agriculture. 8th
Edition. December 2015
www.health.gov/dietaryguidelines/2015/guidelines/

"Dietary Reference Intake." National Institute of Medicine. 2004
www.iom.edu/Reports/2004/Dietary-Reference-Intakes-Water-
Potassium-Sodium-Chloride-and-Sulfate.asp

"Effects of Blood Alcohol Concentration (BAC)." *Centers for Disease Control
and Prevention*. Centers for Disease Control and Prevention, 13 Jan.
2015.
www.cdc.gov/Motorvehiclesafety/impaired_driving/bac.html

"Exercise." *Clinical Updates in Women's Health Care* XIII.2 (2013). Print.

"Fact Sheet on Stress." NIMH RSS. National Institute of Mental Health, 2015.
www.nimh.nih.gov/health/publications/stress/index.shtml

"History of MBSR." *University of Massachusetts Medical School*. Apr. 2015
www.umassmed.edu/cfm/Stress-Reduction/History-of-MBSR/

"How to Practice Alternate Nostril Breathing in Yoga." *Yogaoutlet.com. 2015.
www.yogaoutlet.com/guides/how-to-practice-alternate-nostril-
breathing-in-yoga/*

"Hydrocodone and Oxycodone Overdose." *Medline Plus.* National Institutes
of Health.
www.nlm.nih.gov/medlineplus/ency/article/007285.htm

"Injury Prevention and Control." Sexual Violence Data Sources. March 2015.
www.cdc.gov/violenceprevention/sexualviolence/

"Iron Deficiency Anemia." - *Mayo Clinic*. Mayo Clinic, Jan. 2014.
www.mayoclinic.org/diseases-conditions/iron-deficiency-
anemia/basics/definition/con-20019327

"The Jed Foundation." - *Coalition to Prevent ADHD Medication Misuse
Launched*. The Jed Foundation, Aug. 2014.
www.jedfoundation.org/about/jed-news/CPAMM-launch

"Nutrition and Healthy Eating." *Water: How Much Should You Drink Every
Day?* Mayo Clinic, Aug. 2014. www.mayoclinic.org/healthy-
lifestyle/nutrition-and-healthy-eating/in-depth/water/art-
20044256

"Nutrition." *ACOG Clinical Updates in Women's Health Care* XIII.3 (2014).

"Nutrition Recommendations for Everyone." *Centers for Disease Control and
Prevention*. Centers for Disease Control and Prevention, 04 Oct.
2012. www.cdc.gov/nutrition/everyone/index.html

"Prescription Drug Abuse." Mayo Clinic. Dec. 2014.
www.mayoclinic.org/diseases-conditions/prescription-drug-
abuse/basics/symptoms/con-20032471

"Reporting of Sexual Violence Incidences." *National Institute of Justice.*
Bureau of Justice Statistics. Oct. 2010.
www.nij.gov/topics/crime/rape-sexual-violence/pages/rape-
notification.aspx

"Responding to Campus Sexual Assault." *Responding to Campus Sexual
Assault.* U.S. Department of Justice. July 2014.
www.justice.gov/ovw/responding-campus-sexual-assault

"A Rising Epidemic on College Campuses: Prescription Drug Abuse." *Clinton
Foundation*. The Clinton Foundation, 2015.
www.clintonfoundation.org/blog/2014/01/12/rising-epidemic-
college-campuses-prescription-drug-abuse

Silber, Earl, Tibbett, Jean. "Self-Esteem: Clinical Assessment and
Measurement Validation." *Psychological Reports.* 1965

Secura, Gina M., Jenifer E. Allsworth, Tessa Madden, Jennifer L. Mullersman, and Jeffrey F. Peipert. "The Contraceptive CHOICE Project: Reducing Barriers to Long-Acting Reversible Contraception." *American Journal of Obstetrics and Gynecology*. U.S. National Library of Medicine, 2013.

"Sexual Behavior, Sexual Attraction, and Sexual Identity in the United States." *National Health Statistics Reports.* Centers for Disease Control and Prevention. Number 36. March. 2011

"Stress Management." *Yoga: Fight Stress and Find Serenity*. Mayo Clinic, Feb. 2015. www.mayoclinic.org/healthy-lifestyle/stress-management/in-depth/yoga/art-20044733

"Teen Pregnancy Prevention: Application of CDC's Evidence Based Contraception Guidance." Division of Reproductive Health Centers for Disease Control and Prevention. Nov. 2013. www.cdc.gov/reproductivehealth/UnintendedPregnancy/PDF/TeenPregnancy_SlideSet.PDF

Testa, Maria. "Naturally Occurring Changes in Women's Drinking From High School to College." J of Studies on Alcohol and Drugs 73(2012): 26-33. www.ncbi.nlm.nih.gov/ppmc/artiles/PMC32377009/

"Urinary Tract Infections." American College of Obstetrics and Gynecology FAQ 050 (2011). www.acog.org/Patients/FAQs/Urinary-Tract-Infections-UTIs

"Vaginitis." American College of Obstetrics and Gynecology FAQ 028th ser. (2011). www.acog.org/Patients/FAQs/Vaginitis"Women's Health Care Physicians."

"What is Xanax?" *Drugs.com. 2015. www.drugs.com/xanax.html*

"Women's Health: Eating Disorders." *Office on Women's Health.* U.S. Dept. of Health and Human Services. Sept. 2010. www.womenshealth.gov/body-image/eating-disorders/

Index

H

Handling Difficult Situations
    Learn to Not React, 196
    Sentences, 17, 96, 153, 197
Healthy Food
    Healthy Foods Lists, 31-35
    Late Night Eating, 43
Healthy Target Weight Range
    BMI Calculator, 38
    BMI Chart, 38
    Strategy to Avoid Gaining Weight, 39-40

I

Infections
    Bladder, 67-70
    Products that Mimic Yeast Infections, 66
    Yeast, 65-66
    Urinary Tract, *see bladder*
Iron, 79

M

Mistakes
    How to Move Forward, 193-194
    You Will Not Be Perfect, 193
Mindfulness, 176

N

Nutrition, 21-35, 37-44, 79

P

Prescription Drugs
    Adderall, 167-169
    Oxycontin, 167-168, 170
    Statistics, 167
    Valium, 167-168, 171
    Vyvanse, 167-170

    What to do if Someone Asks/Offers Meds, 168
    Xanax, 167-168, 171
Periods
    Abnormal, 71-75
    Absent, *see Anovulation or Amenorrhea*
    Amenorrhea, 72
    Cramps, *see Dysmenorrhea*
    Dysmenorrhea,
    Gynecologic Conditions, *see Gynecologic Conditions*
    Heavy, *see Menorrhagia*
    Menorrhagia, 71-72
    Metrorrhagia, 72
    Oligomenorrhea, 72
    Tracker, 72, 207

S

Self-Defense
    Courses, 55, 161, 163-164
    Three Steps for, 161-163
Self-Esteem
    Boost, 199-201
    Recognize Your Success, 199-200
    and Sexuality, 93
Sentences, Suggested, 17-18, 96, 138, 168, 189-190, 197
Service to Others, 76, 128, 146
Sex
    Basic Facts, 91-92
    Choosing a Partner, 92, 94
    Dating, 94
    Feeling Empowered, 95
    Oral, 95
    and Self-Esteem, 93
    Suggested Sentences, 96
    What to Do if You Change Your Mind, 96

32862010R00130

Made in the USA
San Bernardino, CA
17 April 2016